Insights on Death & Dying

Joy Ufema, RN, MS

Lippincott Williams & Wilkins
a Wolters Kluwer business
Philadelphia · Baltimore · New York · London
Buenos Aires · Hong Kong · Sydney · Tokyo

STAFF

Executive Publisher
Judith A. Schilling McCann,
RN, MSN

Editorial Director
H. Nancy Holmes

Senior Art Director
Arlene Putterman

Editorial Project Manager
Ann Houska

Copy Editors
Kimberly Bilotta
(supervisor), Scotti Cohn,
Pamela Wingrod

Designer
Debra Moloshok

Illustrator
Judy Newhouse

Cover Design
BJ Crim

Cover Photograph
Daisuke Morita/Photodisc
Green/Getty Images

**Digital Composition
Services**
Diane Paluba (manager),
Joyce Rossi Biletz,
Donna S. Morris

Manufacturing
Beth J. Welsh

Editorial Assistants
Megan L. Aldinger,
Karen J. Kirk, Linda K. Ruhf

Design Assistant
Georg W. Purvis IV

Indexer
Ellen S. Brennan

The articles in this book originally appeared in *Nursing* journal.

The clinical treatments described and recommended in this publication are based on research and consultation with nursing, medical, and legal authorities. To the best of our knowledge, these procedures reflect currently accepted practice. Nevertheless, they can't be considered absolute and universal recommendations. For individual applications, all recommendations must be considered in light of the patient's clinical condition and, before administration of new or infrequently used drugs, in light of the latest package insert information. The authors and publisher disclaim any responsibility for any adverse effects resulting from the suggested procedures, from any undetected errors, or from the reader's misunderstanding of the text.

IDD 010406

Library of Congress
Cataloging-in-Publication Data
Ufema, Joy.
    Insights on death & dying / Joy Ufema.
        p. ; cm.
    "The articles in this book originally appeared in Nursing" —T.p. verso.
    Includes index.
    1. Death. 2. Terminal care. 3. Thanatology.
4. Nursing.
    I. Nursing. II. Title. III. Title: Insights on death
and dying.
    [DNLM: 1. Nursing Care — methods —
Collected Works. 2. Terminal Care — methods —
Collected Works.   WY 152 U23i 2007]
    R726.U34 2007
    616'.029 — dc22
    ISBN 1-58255-973-2 (alk. paper)   2006001162

Contents

Foreword

Joy Ufema has always been ahead of her time. In 1987, when she began writing for *Nursing*, she had already been working in hospice care for 14 years. By sharing her experiences with nurses, she taught us how we could better communicate with and comfort dying patients. In those days, her honest, open approach was revolutionary.

The article she published in *Nursing87* was called "How to Talk to Dying Patients." It starts with a nurse speaking these simple words: "I'm afraid I'll say the wrong thing." The feeling, then and now, is universal — we've all been there. Even after years of experience, many nurses hesitate to discuss death and dying with patients. Yet, more than anything, we want to be the best nurses we can be for our patients and their families at this important time. Joy's advice — be kind, be real, be honest, be yourself — struck a chord with readers hungry for guidance and support.

So the next year, we launched Joy's column, *Insights on Death & Dying*, and it has appeared monthly ever since. Year after year, it has remained one of our most highly read columns. It has "legs" because Joy tells the story of her experiences in a way any nurse can relate to. Setting the scene with dialogue and intimate details, she draws you to the bedside with her. You are there when a dying patient asks Joy the tough questions. You are there as she responds. That's what makes Joy's writing powerful, memorable, and a great learning experience.

Caring for dying patients is like nothing else you do as a nurse. You can't scan the Internet for a formula or algorithm or nursing diagnosis to guide your decisions or help you choose the "right" words. Each patient has different needs, and each of us brings something different to the bedside. Joy lets us know when we need to get rid of our own baggage to do a better job for our patients.

Joy has shared her most moving experiences with *Nursing*'s readers for almost 20 years, and we regularly hear from grateful nurses who have been helped by her work. Now we're proud to bring you this collection of her favorite columns.

Whether or not you're already acquainted with Joy's work, you're in for a treat. Reading Joy's columns is like talking to a friend. She's kind, she's real, and she's always herself.

Cheryl L. Mee, RN,BC, CMSRN, MSN
Editor-In-Chief, *Nursing2006*
Program Director, Nursing2006 Symposium
Lippincott Williams & Wilkins
Philadelphia

Preface

IT WAS ONE of those delicious summer days made all the
more intoxicating because I was 10 years old and had a wood-
shed of raw material at my feet.

"Hey, look at this old box," I said excitedly to my chums. "It
looks like a strongbox for a gold shipment! I've got an idea!
Let's build a stagecoach!"

Thirty years later I was sitting in front of the Director of
Nurses at Harrisburg Hospital relating how I found that my
dying patients didn't require sleeping pills if I spent some time
asking if they would like to share their feelings. "I've got an
idea! I've been attending all these Kübler-Ross seminars,
so let's create a position of Nurse-Specialist in Death and
Dying!"

A decade later, I had received some gracious notoriety for
the experiences gained from that idea. *Nursing* journal asked
that I review and write some articles on death and dying.

Feeling emboldened by those successes, I called *Nursing* and
said, "I've got an idea! Perhaps I could share a portion of my
knowledge in the format of a question-and-response column!"

That was 1986, and I'm honored that my column has appeared in many, many issues since.

Rather than save the entire magazine I began cutting out
those monthly columns, with their beautiful illustrations, and
placing them in plastic sleeves within a three-ring binder.
Amazed by the plethora and diversity of information that had
accumulated over the years, I again telephoned *Nursing* and
said, "I've got an idea! Let's make a little book of my favorite
columns!"

And that is how you came to have this "idea" in your hands at this moment.

But perhaps *why* is more important.

My intention in compiling this assemblage is to offer the reader an opportunity to revisit some of those patients who had an impact on my practice. Those newly introduced to my column may possibly discover a new or different approach in helping the distressed patient and his family.

It is also my desire to impart a bit of practicality to help the nurse feel more comfortable in applying some of the recommendations. I'm not an expert. I have simply chosen to have thousands of experiences with death. Each patient was a teacher, good or bad, in his own right. I want to pass down what I have learned before I "pass on."

Hopefully, these stories will prove beneficial in your professional or personal life. The chapter on "Advocating for patients and families" may be just the key you need when seeking inspiration to take a stand on truth-telling. "Mastering patient management" could provide a few "tricks" to help your father-in-law with severe shortness of breath. I'm emphatic about each of us expressing our own authenticity. "Taking care of yourself" may inspire you to play as hard as you work.

It all comes down to acknowledging that it matters more how we die than that we die. And I believe strongly that we die the way we live. Someone who has been a man of few words all his life will not suddenly become loquacious when told he has inoperable pancreatic cancer. How to help him express those feelings? What do you say when he says, "Tell me the truth, nurse, am I going to die?" And even though each of us will die, it would be trite to say so at that tender moment.

In the rich writing of Larry McMurtry's *Comanche Moon*, we travel into south Texas in the mid 1860s. Two life-long pards, Augustus McCray and Woodrow Cull, have been made Captains of the Rangers. Fighting to tame the West, they have seen an inordinate amount of violence and death. Through it all, their friendship is forged as they've had to protect the men under their command as well as each other.

McCray is seated by the bed of his mortally ill young wife. The hotel room is dirty and sparsely furnished. He gently wipes the sick woman's face with a damp handkerchief.

Captain Cull knocks softly, then tells McCray they've been beckoned by the Governor.

"Woodrow, I can't leave to see no Governor right now. I'm helpin' Nellie die."

Isn't it fortunate that in 2005 we have so much more to offer our dying patients than a cold cloth?

But words are equally important in that repertory of analgesics, antiemetics, and anxiolytics.

Take these words; make them yours, if you so choose. But always find it a noble thing to sit and "help Nellie die."

Joy Ufema, RN, MS

To Rose Foltz,
whose kindness and skill at wordsmithing
make me look good.

I want to offer a special recognition
to the thousands of dear patients and their families
who permitted me to enter their lives during difficult days.
It is from them that these stories come to teach us all
the *arte* and *crafte* of dying.

And
to Linda Lighty,
who patiently typed many columns over the years
on those days when I returned home weary and woeful.
Thank you for always giving me tea by the fire.

Overview

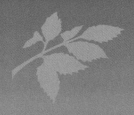

Brief history of end-of-life care

The wife of a rich businessman has contracted tuberculosis. The doctors have pronounced her condition hopeless. The moment has come when she has to be told. There is no question of avoiding it, if only to allow her to make her "final arrangements." But the husband refuses "to tell her about her condition" because, he says, "it would kill her...no matter what happens, it is not I who will tell her." The mother of the dying woman is also reluctant. As for the dying woman, she talks about nothing but new treatments; she seems to be clinging to life, and everyone is afraid of her reaction. However, something has to be done. Finally, the family enlists an old cousin, a poor relation, a mercenary person who throws herself into the task. "Sitting beside the sick woman, she attempts by a skillfully maneuvered conversation to prepare her for the idea of death." But the sick woman suddenly interrupts her, saying, "Ah, my dear! Don't try to prepare me. Don't treat me like a child. I know everything. I know that I haven't much longer to live."

Fast-forward from this 1859 excerpt from Tolstoy's "Three Deaths" cited in Philippe Ariès's tome *The Hour of Our Death* (Knopf, 1981) to one from *A Few Months to Live: Different Paths to Life's End,* a publication by Staton, Shuy, and Byock (Georgetown University Press, 2001):

"My doctor seemed to want to be encouraging as opposed to discouraging. I think maybe he personally made the decision about whether I could handle the [knowledge]. A lot of that is a blur with what I was told. I know that I remember my husband coming in, and he was in so much despair. I was asking him to talk to me and tell me and that's when he started crying and saying, 'I don't want to lose you. I don't know if I can handle this.'"

In 1973 at the Royal Victoria Hospital in Montreal, Dr. Bal Mount and colleagues conducted a study in which physicians were found to be reluctant to be candid about death and dying, yet the patients wanted honest, open discussion.

As reflected in the above pieces of literature and reinforced by the Royal Victoria study, death is seen as the enemy except by those doing the dying.

We used to see death as a natural consequence of life. In fact, by the 1500s the *Ars Moriendi* tradition was prevalent. Translated as "the arte and crafte of dying," these guidebooks described rituals that were to be performed as part of the deathbed scene.

The "main character" wasn't the dying man himself, but the priest. It was he who gave guidance in proper leave-taking, the giving away of chattel, and the dutiful goodbye. The patient then assumed a reclining position and waited for death to arrive.

By the end of World War II however, the bedroom was replaced by the hospital ward and, logically, the priest by the physician. With the more technical advances came a new concept: the failed machine.

The personal relationship between doctor and patient became altered. This depersonalization was tolerable if the treatments resulted in cure. But it wasn't as easily endured if death was a more likely prospect.

So we now have death = failure = denial.

Fortunately, the early 1960s saw the prevalence of writings, lectures, and seminars on death and dying.

Most eminent at the time was the ground-breaking work of Elisabeth Kübler-Ross, the Swiss psychiatrist who wrote *On Death and Dying*. Her observations, after interviewing hundreds of terminally ill patients, proposed the five stages commonly experienced: Denial, Anger, Bargaining, Depression and, finally, Acceptance.

This instant best-seller brought death "out of the closet," although some thanatologists felt it was a cookbook "recipe" that labeled patients. I acknowledge the value of Dr. Kübler-Ross's contribution but recall shuddering at seeing a freshly scrubbed student nurse, clutching a copy of the book, striding determinedly down the hall, seeking an unsuspecting patient upon whom to affix one of the five steps in the complex journey of leaving the planet Earth.

The first free-standing, bricks-and-mortar hospice was built in New Haven, Connecticut, in 1974. It was a prototype based on Saint Christopher's Hospice in Sydenham, outside of London. Its founder, Dame Cicely Saunders, a social worker turned nurse turned physician, summed up the philosophy of palliative care by stating, "The patient should be in the center."

Does that wisdom still hold true in how end-of-life care is practiced today?

The current thinking

There's an ancient Persian legend that tells of the servant who burst into his master's quarters pleading for a fast horse to flee to Samarra. He explained that he had just met Death while walking in the marketplace in Baghdad. The master granted the servant's request. Later, while walking in the marketplace the master met Death sitting near a tree. "Why did you frighten my servant?" inquired the master. Death replied, "I did not wish to frighten him. I was a bit surprised to see him here for I have an appointment with him later tonight in Samarra."

And so, no matter how fast the horse, each of us has an appointment with Death.

The problem is, we don't really believe that we will die. If we did, we certainly would live our lives differently.

Contributing to this denial is the influence of the media. Spend an hour or two watching such television shows as "ER" and "House." The prevailing message is when it comes to saving a life, the end always justifies the means. And even if Death is the victor, the fight was worth the price of dignity!

Even in the midst of futility lies a sense of entitlement to have "everything" done that can be done. And even if the unfortunate patient ends up being in a persistent vegetative state, like 25,000 today in this country, he can be fed through tubes and pee through tubes...but, hey! He didn't die!

Years ago, if a man didn't come in from the fields to eat dinner, his son or daughter was sent to fetch him. There the farmer lay, dead from a myocardial infarction, face down in the sweet earth he tenderly plowed. The team of horses stood quietly, waiting for his familiar commands. Later, they would be asked to pull the wagon bearing the farmer's coffin to the family cemetery. It was all so lovingly natural.

Now, I find the modern hospital death obscene. I'm offended by the absence of decency that every human deserves.

"You wanted us to do everything we could! Now look what we've got!" I want to shout.

Don't people know there are worse things than death?

This is the time to utilize one of the 2,400 hospice home care programs in the nation. Most provide an excellent service at helping families grant the requests of patients to die at home.

The problem is that 37% of patients die within 7 days of admission. This hardly affords time for the hospice team to get to know the patient and family. It's difficult to advocate for how the patient defines a meaningful death when he's comatose during the admission process.

If the physician feels the time to discuss palliative care has arrived, and if she's comfortable in initiating the conversation, the patient might thwart those efforts by saying, "But Doctor, I'm not ready for hospice." Which really means, "I'm not ready to die. Isn't there something more you can do?"

One hundred years ago, the town doctor sat on an old rocking chair beside the tiny bed on which a feverish child lay. He gave laudanum and cooling baths. As the terrified parents stood in the lamplight, surely they wished for the physician to "do more." But he had nothing more, and the child died.

Today, not only do we have more, we may have too much in our arsenal in the war on death. A 90-year-old lady is taken from the nursing home to the hospital, where aspiration pneumonia is easily diagnosed. The poor dear is frail and has lived long enough to develop congestive heart failure and some mild dementia.

Insertion of a feeding tube is recommended. The daughter is hesitant until the attending physician defines the procedure as "minor" and then adds, "You wouldn't want your mother to starve, now, would you?"

The social worker or nurse offers the option of "just keeping mother comfortable." There is no advance directive because we don't really believe we're going to die, and now the daughter is feeling confused and fearful.

"I don't want to be responsible for killing her."

I'm fairly certain that aspiration pneumonia occurred 100 years ago. Because we didn't have feeding tubes then, none were offered. The patient knew he was going to die, as did his family and physician.

This focus in the 21st Century of keeping the organism alive is becoming distasteful.

Because death is the only sure thing we know will happen one day, why aren't we preparing ourselves for the event?

"If I'd known I was going to live this long, I'd have taken better care of myself."

I fear for our society in general and for healthcare providers in particular.

Betty Ferrell conducted a survey at the City of Hope Medical Center. Of the nurses polled, 66% rated care of the dying better in 2000 than 5 years earlier. But the survey revealed that, overall, nurses felt their basic education to be inadequate in preparing for end-of-life care. They're distressed by patients experiencing unrelieved pain and symptoms.

These feelings are further substantiated in the audiences throughout the country to whom I speak on my lecture circuit. Nurses are frustrated by not knowing what to say and fear "saying the wrong thing." They're confused and exhausted by providing care in the midst of futility. They feel guilty for inflicting fruitless treatments, even when the patient himself requests it. They're finding it difficult to receive intrinsic rewards.

End-of-life care guidelines
For the patient

Just as a hand massaged in an uncomfortable position remains uncomfortable after the massage, a patient lying in sweat-soaked linens while being counseled about dying isn't benefiting from the counsel.

The most important thing for a nurse to do for a dying patient is to be his nurse! By that I mean wash his achy body and sweaty hair, massage his back and smooth his sheets, give superb and thorough mouth care, and then sit by his side.

We know patients fear pain and abandonment, yet we could do so much more in both areas.

The following five points identified as equating quality of care at the end of life may provide guidance.

#1 To receive adequate pain and symptom control

It's obvious if the patient is an "8" on the pain scale of 0 to 10 that he won't and can't fully enjoy a visit from his exuberant, loquacious 5-year-old granddaughter.

Nor can the young mother with ovarian cancer suffering with intractable nausea from a partial bowel obstruction speak of her fears of leaving twin sons.

We owe the terminally ill person the commitment of working indefatigably to provide aggressive palliative care.

There's a difference between the biology of disease and the experience of illness. When the patient is upset, he has more symptoms. Therefore, the logical thing to do is validate his feelings and concerns.

The French philosopher Simone Weil once said that the only suitable question to ask another human being was "What are you going through?" A gentle touch on the dying person's shoulder and a sincere, "I can't imagine how difficult this must be for you," tells the patient you are not only listening but are actually hearing his concerns.

The chapter titled "Mastering patient management" offers specifics on treating dyspnea, constipation, bone pain, and much more.

#2 To avoid the inappropriate prolongation of life

I stood beside the oncologist, nudging him gently toward the head of the bed. The patient was a 72-year-old gentleman, retired from teaching at the local junior high school. The cancer of his jaw and chin had been particularly menacing. Now, with further treatment not a favorable option, hospice was to be offered.

"The chemo isn't really working," the doctor explained.

The patient nodded almost imperceptibly.

Breaking the uncomfortable silence, the doctor blurted out, "But we could give you more, if you want."

Mr. Shaeffer didn't want.

He might have wanted his physician to be replaced by Richard Parker, who might have explained the end of life as he wrote in the January 2002 *Annals of Internal Medicine:* "I liken the process to a clock no longer wound every day that gradually runs out of energy. When the clock runs down, all the parts stop."

It's important to the dying person that he not be kept sicker, longer. Prolonging life simply to stave off death one more day wastes precious time during which the patient's energy and the opportunity to come to terms with himself can be lost.

These cherished days can otherwise be spent with loving family and friends, like a king leaving a banquet table.

Diagnosed with a deadly form of leukemia, Stuart Alsop quipped, "Just as a sleepy man must lie down to sleep so must a dying man lie down to die."

#3 To feel a sense of control

Derek Doyle, my hero and esteemed palliative care physician from Edinburgh, Scotland, tells of the terminally ill patient hesitant to be admitted to the hospice. She asks, "Do I have to eat?"

The soft response, "No."

"Do I have to wash?"

Again, "No."

"May I sleep as long as I want?"

"Yes."

Her cancer was out of control. Her emotions were barely under control. Now, she has this opportunity to regain a semblance of control in her life, something each of us takes for granted. The moment we get out of bed in the morning, we take control of the events of the day. We eat anything we want for breakfast and it stays down. We run upstairs to retrieve a sweater and we aren't dropped to our knees by pain. Our body is still our servant.

But the body of Dr. Doyle's patient has betrayed her, and she seeks control in the simplest ways because to ask for more is risky.

I recall caring for a lovely lady with a difficult, aloof husband. When she had her mastectomy, at first he was fairly attentive, but as she regained a modicum of strength he withdrew. Even when lung and bone metastasis forced her to take to her bed, he would immediately retreat after complying with a request.

While visiting, I observed her ask her husband to bring her some fresh water.

"And, John, make sure you put two or three ice cubes in, not too many."

Silence from the kitchen.

"And, John, would you please put it in the blue glass?"

She hadn't had much control in the marriage, but her terminal condition provided both the bravery and the permission to make requests.

She didn't push it by asking John to give her a backrub.

It's imperative to be acutely aware of ways to give the patient a sense of control in an uncontrollable situation. Patients want to feel worthy of being served, not patronized. You wouldn't want to attempt to provide control by saying, "Would you like your bath before or after your favorite television show?" This is a tactic useful in pediatrics, but your patient is an adult who has made major decisions for herself all her life.

It's much more dignified to ask if she would like to be bathed and, if so, when would be best for her.

Keep in mind, she's losing all the sunsets, all of her grandbabies, all of her music and books, all of her all.

So, when, not if, she's pushing the call button every few minutes, she isn't doing it to harass you. She's simply attempting to regain some control in her world. You have control over yours. Be kind and compassionate.

#4 To relieve the personal burden on family

It's difficult to lie around. It's even more troublesome to always be on the receiving end of a relationship. To be lovingly cared for may be comforting; to be taken care of may be demeaning.

The hospice home care philosophy states "the patient and family is the unit of care." Yet, we may be asking a young family member to have her first death experience be that of a beloved parent, brother, or child.

Granted, if given a choice, most people prefer to die at home, cared for by family and friends in familiar surroundings. In fact, 90% of Americans feel the family has the responsibility to provide care at the end of life.

But for the patient to see exhaustion and fear in the eyes of his caregivers can have an effect on the quality of leave-taking. Perhaps he's a husband and father. His role had always been to protect his "girls." Now he sees his wife and daughters struggling to keep up with the washing, the cooking, and the caring. They fall asleep after sitting down for a few minutes. This caretaker fatigue may give an unspoken message of "burden."

I'm most impressed when a hospice team member helps organize a list of volunteers, staff, and family with dates and times of visits. The patient can be informed of the schedule and may feel less of a burden knowing his grieving family is relieved of the 24-hour care-giving duty.

It's valuable to determine how deeply the family feels they are being cared for. As mentioned previously, French philosopher Simone Weil said that the only suitable question to ask another human being was, "What are you going through?" This inquiry must be posed and the response clearly heard if we are to really call the patient's family our "patient," too.

What better gift to the dying man than to see his household being cared for as well as they give care to him. By acknowledging, "you all are doing a good job in a difficult situation," we may see how a bit of genuine praise can rejuvenate.

#5 To strengthen relationships with loved ones

Fulfilling this particular end-of-life need by the patient can be paradoxical. In strengthening relationships with those he loves, the dying man may find it harder to say goodbye.

"I never knew I was loved so much by my son. Now I wish I had more time to enjoy it."

But because it matters more how we die than that we die, it's better to die being loved.

Ralph Waldo Emerson said, "For every minute you are angry, you lose sixty seconds of happiness."

At the end of life, when time is measured in minutes, there's an urgency to bring any and all whom the patient wants to his deathbed. He needs to say "Thank you," "Please forgive me," "I forgive you," "I love you," and "Goodbye." And he needs each person to acknowledge those words of declaration. But illness and death can cause family members to cope by withdrawing. These "short and sweet" statements are the perfect tools to provide anxious loved ones the means to finish a relationship.

As they see the value in last words, some families may want to take the conversation to a deeper level by asking the patient, "What's the one thing you want us to remember about you?"

My own father fell dead from mitral stenosis onto the shop floor where he worked for the Pennsylvania Railroad. Reticent, he never spoke about himself much, leaving me to wonder about his unfulfilled hopes and dreams. But during the viewing of his 42-year-old body, I recall shaking the grease-stained hands of men who, one after another, told me what a skillful wheel mechanic he was.

This newfound knowledge comforted me through the many sad days and weeks to follow.

By hearing how one would like to be remembered, survivors share something special and can honor that life by reminding each other of their loved one's self-identity.

Who's most important to the palliative care patient? Family. But it isn't until he sees his clan unified and supportive of each other as they stand around his bed that he can finally lie back, sigh, and rest in peace.

For the caregiver

To a youngster dreaming of being a nurse, that aspiration usually evokes images of healing people, helping them to get well and return to normalcy. I doubt there's even a remote consideration that, at some point, healing and helping won't be enough and death will enter to steal away any semblance of normalcy.

The new nurse will be unpleasantly surprised at the disparity between the way people die and the way they want to die.

And so, just as we would "arm" her with protective gear to care for a patient with bacterial meningitis, we owe her the right "equipment" to provide end-of-life care.

First, I would remind her to be kind. This may sound trivial but the terminally ill individual puts up an antenna that quickly scans for signals of "compassion," "kindness," and "sincerity."

If these qualities are absent or blocked by fear, he'll be considerate and civil. But he won't be sharing anything.

Kindness isn't what you do or say; rather, it's how you are fully present with another.

The patient can sense whether or not you want to be with him. It's infinitely rewarding to do so.

Second, the nurse providing end-of-life care needs to listen with the heart. It isn't about telling or not telling a diagnosis and prognosis. It's about listening to the patient's concerns.

In the chapter "Communicating effectively" are several examples on how to enhance those listening skills.

As the nurse gains more experience, she'll begin to discern that the terminally ill individual has five facets of dying. They are spiritual, physical, social, financial, and psychological. These divisions may require specialists to help the patient resolve unique needs. The nurse doesn't have to know everything about each area but to know when to ask for help. The woman worried about a punitive God needs a sensitive clergyperson, while the gentleman who has no insurance needs to speak with a knowledgeable social worker.

Don't try to be all things to all people.

Do what you do, well.

Patients and family find comfort and security in a competent nurse.

Our nurse would want to be knowledgeable about advance directives and their application. If a patient is admitted repeatedly, his advance directive needs to be retrieved from Medical Records and placed in his current chart. It isn't necessary to discuss the contents but simply to ask, "Do you still want to abide by your directive?" This sends a clear message that the nurse respects the serious consideration required for this individual to put in writing his wishes regarding matters of life and death.

She may have difficulty with some physicians who disregard the legality of an advance directive and defer decision-making from a competent patient to a family member. This usually occurs when the patient makes a decision unpopular with the physician.

Then there will be physicians who delay writing "Do Not Resuscitate" because of irrational fears the nurse will translate that order to "Do Nothing." Perhaps the nurse could provide a copy of the American Nurses Association Code of Ethics for the physician's perusal. It's handed out at most orientation programs and frequently found on bulletin boards at the nurse's station. She might place an asterisk beside provision #2 which states, "The nurse's primary commitment is to the patient, whether an individual, family, group, or community."

I would also want to arm this nurse with the option of utilizing the hospital ethics committee. Those members are skilled at discussing dilemmas and helping discern what's best for the patient, not his family, or his preacher, or his long-lost niece from Arizona. Questions asked in the context of "burden or benefit" help decipher the moral predicaments that seem more prevalent in a population living longer and developing several chronic diseases.

It's worthy of the professional nurse to advocate for the dying. She needs to trust her experience and instincts to know when to suggest "comfort care only." Again, this doesn't mean "Do not provide any care." It's at this time in the trajectory of serious illness that the word "aggressive palliative care" applies.

The goal is to meliorate all distressing symptoms.

Specific hints found in the chapter "Mastering patient management" will provide effective results in this challenging area.

Last, it's never true to say there's nothing more to be done. As you are leaving the deathbed, turn around, look, and see your patient. Is she better from your care than she was before your visit?

.1.
Communicating effectively

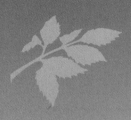

Being there at the end

Years ago I had a home health care patient who was recovering from triple bypass surgery. His family always kept in touch with me through cards and occasional phone calls. We felt like one big family. Yesterday, the patient's daughter called to tell me that her father had suffered a stroke and isn't expected to live. She didn't ask me to visit, and I didn't think to offer. But now I'm wondering if it would be appropriate for me to see him before he dies. What do you think? —R.Y., *Delaware*

JUST DO IT!

After all, the daughter might have been afraid to ask you to visit her dad, thinking you'd be too busy and might say no. Her call was a subtle way of saying "You helped before. Could you please help again?"

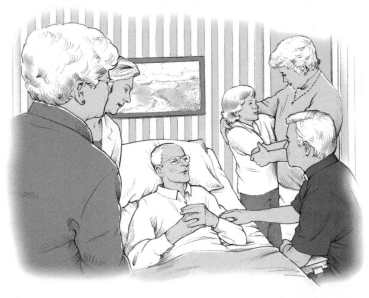

Also, you've had a special, ongoing relationship with this patient and his family. So being included in his dying process would be very appropriate.

Never underestimate the value of your presence at the deathbed. A hundred or so years ago, a dying person would "take to his bed" and summon friends, family, and clergy. During this gathering, he gave away all of his belongings. And there, with dignity, surrounded by loved ones, he was watched over until death finally came.

When one of my patients, Barney, was dying, family, friends, and past acquaintances arrived to show their love and support. An ex-girlfriend read psalms to him as she wept softly. Fellow Alcoholics Anonymous members told stories of how often Barney had rescued them at 2 a.m., when they'd called in desperation. And one of his childhood friends, who'd waited hours on standby for a flight, got the chance to stand by his pal one final time.

They came because he was dying—to honor his years of living. That kind of caring is always welcome. ✍

Helping hand

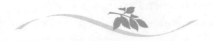

My next-door neighbor was recently diagnosed with cancer. He's back home after being hospitalized for several weeks, and I'd like to do something to help him out. The problem is I'm not sure what to do or say. Can you help? — C.B., Quebec

I'M GLAD TO HEAR that you're concerned about your neighbor and want to help him. Too often, people are paralyzed by fear and avoid close contact with those who have cancer.

I suggest that you call him before visiting. If he's experiencing adverse reactions to chemotherapy, he may not want company. And you should recognize that he has the right to say so. (Although well-meaning, some visitors are offended if they aren't enthusiastically received.)

That doesn't mean he wouldn't appreciate your telephone calls. Many patients have told me they love to talk on the phone because they can stay in bed without feeling obligated to get dressed and "made up." In fact, those who live alone like a daily call at a scheduled time. That way, they know someone will be checking in.

You might also send your neighbor cards with little notes. He can read and reread them at his leisure.

Be careful about sending flowers, though. Chemotherapy can affect the sense of smell, so the fragrance of flowers could actually be unpleasant. A plant would be a better choice.

Food is a big issue. During one of your visits or phone calls, ask your neighbor what he feels like having. If he wants gelatin, don't take him a big, fat chocolate cake. And make sure you find out what flavor of gelatin he wants.

I also have a few thoughts about "what to say."

Don't worry about being profound. Just be yourself. Let him know that you're thinking about him. One patient told me that weeks after her course of chemotherapy ended, friends said to her, "Oh, Gwen, we thought about you so much." She wished they'd told her that back when she needed them.

Subconsciously, you may be reluctant to visit because you're suntanned and feeling good. You have a right to be happy and healthy. So does your neighbor. But right now, he isn't whole.

The best you can give him is *your* wholeness: your smile, your laugh, your heart, and your spirit.

Talk about the same things you talked about before. Let him know that you're willing to discuss anything — including how he feels about having cancer.

Relax. And be real. ✎

In the driver's seat

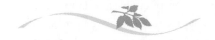

Recently, I was assigned to care for a terminally ill man who told me he no longer felt valuable as a husband. He's too weak to work or even to do odd jobs around the house and knows he'll never regain his strength. What can I say to him?
—*R.M., New Hampshire*

THE LOSS OF A meaningful role would depress anyone. Many of us identify ourselves, perhaps falsely, by our jobs. Imagine someone saying, "You know the work you love to do? Well, you can't ever do it again." That's the kind of thief dying is.

But people can continue to find meaning in their lives, even if their accustomed roles change—a lesson I learned from Tony and Angela.

Tony was terminally ill with lung cancer. I'd met him and his wife when he was hospitalized for treatment, and they took a liking to me. When Tony was discharged, Angela invited me to their home for dinner.

As I stood outside the door on the appointed night, I could hear a commotion inside. Hesitantly, I rang the bell, and the door swung open. Seeing me, Angela burst into laughter and hugged me.

"Joy! Joy! So good you here! You can talk sense to this man."

Tony was sitting up in the rumpled bed, his eyes lit with intensity.

"He won't let me learn to drive!" said Angela, gesturing wildly.

The arguing continued briefly, both parties appealing for support. Careful to remain neutral, I focused on my patient, who was now severely short of breath. I helped him lie back and increased his oxygen flow.

"Please just rest and try to get your breathing slowed," I said softly. Ten minutes later they both were calmer. Angela sat on the bed and I pulled up a chair.

"Now, I think I might have a solution. Tony, I know you've always been a protector for Angela. How would you both feel about my getting a driver's education book from the department of motor vehicles?" Turing to Angela, I said, "Tony can help teach you the rules and we could get a special friend like me, to help you learn to drive."

"Tony, you be my teach," Angela agreed. "You a good teach."

"Why don't you want Angela to drive?" I asked Tony.

He said, "I know she gonna need to drive after I'm gone. I just no want her to be away from me now."

Angela's eyes filled with tears. "Oh my Tony. Not now. After. Then is it okay if Joy helps?"

"Yeah, after. But now I teach you with the book. I be you teach."

Like Tony, your patient wants to continue protecting in the way he feels worthwhile. Perhaps you could find one of those home fix-it books so he can be her "teach" for "after." ≈

Collections of a lifetime

In our busy medical/surgical unit, we nurses typically care for patients who are moderately to acutely ill. We do our best to cover for each other if a terminally ill patient needs extra time to talk. While we're comfortable being good listeners, we'd also like to know the right questions to ask. Any suggestions?
— *B.D., Tennessee*

KUDOS TO YOU and your colleagues for choosing to participate in these important conversations. Many health care professionals see death as the enemy and spend lots of energy trying to avoid it. Sadly, they miss out on the chance for a memorable and unique experience with a fellow mortal.

Rather than focusing on the "right" questions to ask, I'd advise you to listen with undivided attention, then respond appropriately. I usually begin by introducing myself and telling the patient about my role. For example: "Mrs. Jansen, I'm a nurse specialist and I work with patients who are seriously ill. Would you like to talk about how things are going for you?"

This approach is forthright and specific. Now she knows I'm a nurse — someone who could provide physical care if needed — and she knows I'm aware that she's seriously ill. (Most patients prefer that term to "terminally ill.") Mrs. Jansen also knows that I'm willing to talk about a subject that many people avoid. And I've given her control, allowing her to choose whether or not to talk. She may say no (over the years, only two out of hundreds have preferred not to speak with me), but at least she knows my services were sincerely offered.

If she chooses to talk, I ask permission to sit on the bed and do so gently. I then simply ask, "Is all this getting a bit rough for you?"

Sharing this insight that being seriously ill does get rough often releases a flow of words that have been kept inside amid all those cancer cells. She risks trusting me, then lets her feelings of hope and hopelessness, anger and guilt, fear and pain come out. The sharing is intimate and sacred. My "calling" to work is reinforced, and I'm reminded that I, too, must die.

She may say, "The doctor told me 3 to 6 months." I ask, "Is that good or bad news?" Patients who are "sick and tired" may feel relieved that an omnipotent physician has said this suffering will continue for only a few more months.

Mrs. Jansen replies that she's only 63 and had hoped to live longer. This is a timely opening to explore the values in the life already lived and not yet completed. I ask about things she's accomplished.

Proudly, she tells me of her twin sons. I ask about things of meaning she's leaving behind. She speaks of her collection of salt and pepper shakers, then muses about bequeathing them to her favorite niece. I ask her about her beliefs, in life and afterlife. And I ask if she's suffering. She says no. I touch her near her heart and ask if she's "suffering in her soul." She smiles and says no.

This is what I do and how I do it. All the while, I'm reminded of the lesson I learned from a beautiful white-haired woman. I asked her, "What's the most important thing you would teach me?" She replied, "Be kind. Be kind. Be kind."

Running out of time?

As the charge nurse on the evening shift, I'm frequently assigned several patients. I feel guilty for not having time to sit and talk with those who are terminally ill. Sometimes I want to start a conversation, but I'm afraid I'll be interrupted, so I just let it go. Then I feel even worse. What can I do? —M.E., Maryland

MANY NURSES EXPRESS this same frustration. But don't assume that you need a huge block of time to really talk. When we're fully present, listening, and giving our undivided attention to the patient, we can accomplish more in a few minutes than we would in an hour of quasi-listening. The following case illustrates my point.

The cardiologist had written a consult for me to speak with a man with end-stage heart failure. He wasn't a candidate for transplant and nothing more could be offered him medically.

I entered the room and found Mr. Nestor propped up in bed supported by six well-positioned pillows. He looked tired and pale. A young woman, his granddaughter, sat beside the bed with her hand resting on his arm.

I introduced myself, saying, "My name is Joy, and I'm a nurse. I work with patients who are seriously ill. Do you feel like talking about what you're going through and what help you might need?"

He motioned to the young woman to get his hearing aid, saying, "I want to hear what she has to say."

Once the small amplifier was in place, I said, "Actually, Mr. Nestor, I want to hear what you have to say. Is all this getting a little rough for you?"

He nodded, then said, "I guess Doc Simon told you about my worn-out ticker."

I smiled, nodded, then touched his hand.

"Aw, we all gotta go sometime." He leaned over and kissed his granddaughter on the top of her head. "Karla don't want me to go," he continued, "but it's in God's hands now."

"Mr. Nestor," I said, "there are some things that are in your hands, like where you want to live the rest of your days."

"Well now, I want to go home, if that's possible."

I knew he lived alone so I asked who'd take care of him. With that, Karla stood and announced, "I will. Well, my mom and I will."

Mr. Nestor seemed pleased with this pronouncement and settled back into the pillows, breathing easier, literally and figuratively.

I softly explained about hospice and emphasized our goal of keeping him comfortable.

"This also means that you won't be brought back to the hospital. You'll die at home, surrounded by your wonderful family."

"No, I don't want to come back to the hospital," he panted. "Karla and her mom aren't real flesh and blood, but they've loved me better than my own family."

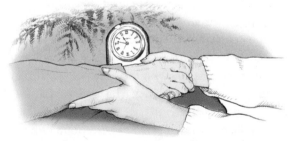

We all sat together, holding hands. The conversation had been one of respectful honesty, direct but tender. And it took about 12 minutes.

I'm not recommending that you try to see how quickly you can achieve this kind of discussion. I'm saying that even within your limited time, you can provide what's most important: your personal attention, fully focused and caring.

Spiritual journeys

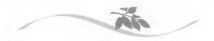

I'm not what you'd call religious, although I've been known to say a prayer with my patients in the dialysis unit. Lately, though, it seems that my patients don't have any religious convictions. They never discuss religion, even when their condition is deteriorating. How can I get them to open up about their religious belief?
—J.S., Illinois

GEORGE BERNARD SHAW SAID, "Religion is a great force — the only real motive force in the world. But you must get at a man through his own religion, not yours."

I think what you're talking about is not religion but spirituality. Your dialysis patients may not all have formal religious convictions, but they may have a spiritual side.

Rather than limiting your focus to religion, I suggest you open a dialogue by asking your patients if they feel like sharing what it's like to be seriously ill. You've probably been working with them long enough to have established a "cushion of caring" — a relationship of trust and an honest exchange of feelings. After all, they trust you with their life's blood. If they sense a genuineness about you, they'll be grateful that you care enough to ask about such an intimate facet of their lives.

You must understand each patient's perception of his situation. So listen from your heart, your spirit — not your religion. There must be no judging or distorting. Just take it from the patient's viewpoint — regardless of the facts! Tell him that it's okay to practice his own comforting spiritual rituals in your unit.

When a sick and dying fellow human being honors you by sharing what's deep in his marrow, you'll know the difference between religion and spirituality.

Right words

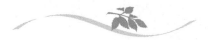

My brother died suddenly of a heart attack. In her grief, his wife told my 7-year-old nephew that God took his father because he was a good man and God wanted him in heaven. I'm afraid the boy will misunderstand that, but I don't know what to say to her. Can you help? — S.K., *New Mexico*

I'M SURE YOUR SISTER-IN-LAW meant well. But I agree that her explanation may confuse your nephew. He may feel angry and resentful toward God — after all, he needs his father more than God does. Also, he may worry that if he's good, God will take him too. Your sister-in-law shouldn't be surprised if he starts misbehaving.

The first thing you can do is sit down and talk with her. Share what I've told you, and offer to help her explain your brother's death to the boy. Avoid criticizing her, though. Even though her words weren't the best, at least she told him about his father's death herself.

When you talk with your nephew, explain that death is a natural part of life. Everything — the flowers, trees, birds, and people — will die. Tell him that some people die when they're young, but most live to be old, like his grandparents. Emphasize that he didn't say or do anything to cause his father's death.

Also, let him know that he may feel sad or strange, but that those feelings are normal. Tell him you feel sad too. Encourage him to talk with you or his mother, even if you both cry.

If the funeral hasn't taken place yet, make sure he's given a chance to attend. You or your sister-in-law might explain what will happen at the funeral, then let him decide whether or not to go.

If he wants to attend, you or another relative should stay beside him. His mother may be too grief-stricken to support him. If he decides against going, make sure he knows that he may visit the grave whenever he wants.

One more thing: Your nephew may react to your talk by going out to play. This isn't because he's insensitive or doesn't understand. Like adults, children use denial as a buffer — it's a perfectly normal response.

Just reassure him that you love him and that you'll be there for him.

In the coming months, you might try to make time to take him fishing or to a baseball game or movie. Something may trigger a comment about his father and start an important conversation about death — and that could make you both feel better.

The toughest question

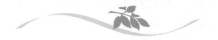

I'm a recent graduate assigned to a medical/surgical unit. My colleagues say this is a good place to get experience, which is what I want. Just one problem: I'm afraid I won't know what to say if a terminally ill patient ask me if he's dying. How do you respond when patients ask you that?—N.L., Massachusetts

FIRST, CONGRATULATIONS on completing your nursing studies. I know you'll find great rewards in this career. And you can't beat the experience you'll get in a medical/surgical unit.

Yes, I've had patients look in my eyes and ask if they're going to die. And I always respond honestly. It's proof of my respect for them. Every now and again, I hear someone respond to a patient's inquiry about death with, "Well, we're all dying." I find this condescending. Of course we're all dying. But unlike our terminally ill patients, we don't awaken each morning and wonder if we'll die *today*.

I remember caring for Art, who arrived in the unit from the ED coughing up bloody, frothy, sputum from his lungs. He was thrashing about in the bed as if an ancient survival reflex had kicked in. Death was imminent, and every cell in his being knew it.

He stared up at me, blood pouring from the corners of his mouth, as I adjusted his I.V. line. "Oh God. Oh, my God! Am I dying?"

I said, "You're very sick, Art, but we're doing everything we can for you. We're all right here with you."

Art closed his eyes and died minutes later.

Another patient I remember was a 64-year-old woman with cancer of the larynx. A lifelong smoker, she'd hold her cigarettes up to her tracheostomy tube to inhale. To communicate,

I spoke and she scribbled on a notepad. In the middle of a "light" conversation, she suddenly wrote across the pad in bold letters, "TELL ME THE TRUTH—AM I DYING?"

I took her hand and looked into her eyes. "Yes, you are," I said. "But you won't be alone, and we'll keep you comfortable." She smiled weakly, squeezed my hand, and mouthed, "Thank you." (I still have that sheet of paper.)

Some patients who have extensive metastases sense that the malignancy is out of control. When they ask, "Am I going to die?" I reply, "It looks like this cancer is getting ahead of us. But we're going to go through this together and treat every symptom to keep you comfortable." I say this because many terminally ill patients fear pain and abandonment more than anything. We need to address these fears head-on.

After you respond honestly to your patient's question about his impending death, be sure to follow up by asking, "Do you feel like talking about what you're going through?" If he doesn't, respect his wishes; he may decide to share his feelings another time. But if he does want to talk, sit down with him, touch his hand or shoulder if you feel comfortable doing that, and give him your undivided attention.

Listen with your heart as well as your ears. You'll do just fine.

Ill at ease

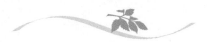

My best friend is dying of breast cancer, and I'm uncomfortable visiting her. I've cared for terminally ill patients at the hospital where I work, but this is different. I don't know what to say when I'm with her. Can you help? — *E.M., Quebec*

YOUR HONESTY IS your greatest asset. Many professionals are unwilling to admit feeling ill at ease in this situation. They end up plunking themselves down at a patient's bedside and working through their own uneasiness at the dying person's expense. Your caring is shining through. All you need are a few guidelines.

First of all, it's okay to be afraid; that's real. Remember: Death affects us. But don't let your fear paralyze you — go visit.

Your friend will sense your anxiety, so be up-front and confess what's on your mind. You might say, "I'm uncomfortable and don't know exactly what to say, but I care about what you're going through."

That simple statement can ease tension and set a tone of openness. Once your friend hears you being "real," she has permission to take the conversation wherever she wants. She may choose not to discuss her death and dying, but she'll know for sure that it would be a safe road to take with you.

What a lovely gift to give your best friend. ✐

When to clam up

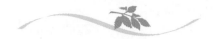

*As a new nurse being oriented to home health care hospice, I
accompanied an experienced nurse to several homes. She had
terrific clinical skills, but her listening skills didn't match up. When
a patient's husband was speaking to her about his wife's condition,
she didn't seem to hear his underlying concerns and fears. She just
kept saying "uh-huh" and "yes, uh-huh" and writing her notes.
When she spoke to him, it was strictly clinical. As we left, I put my
hands on the gentleman's arm. He looked so sad.*

*If I hadn't been riding with this nurse, I would have gone back
in to sit and listen. Would I be out of line to talk with her about
this?* — M.J., *Mississippi*

THE KEY WORD in your question is listen. A physician with
advanced cancer once told a group of medical students, "Give
me just 10 minutes of interested, uninterrupted listening, and
I'll tell you all you need to know to help me." Good advice.
Listening is a skill that's sorely neglected in nursing and medicine alike.

To listen, you must be fully present. That means sitting
down, shutting up, and paying attention with your whole
being. You're not listening when:
+ you're in a hurry
+ you're thinking about yourself
+ you interrupt
+ you ask the same question twice
+ you don't ask any questions
+ you assume you know what the other person's going to say.

Rather than confronting your colleague directly, I suggest
discussing the incident privately with her team leader. Possibly
your colleague wasn't emotionally available that one day for

some personal reason, or she was feeling the pressure of a busy day with other patients to visit. Maybe the next day was different. Unfortunately, patients don't always have another day, and their spouses may be reluctant to reach out to a nurse one more time.

If your colleague consistently demonstrates poor listening skills, speaking to her supervisor allows you to advocate for those who are too overwhelmed to speak for themselves. You might also suggest that she arrange a staff-development session on listening skills for the benefit of all your colleagues. ✍

Panic at 2 a.m.

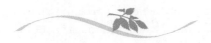

I work as an on-call nurse for a large hospice agency. Recently, several families receiving hospice services panicked at 2 a.m. and called emergency medical services about their terminally ill loved ones. Each of the patients was transported to the hospital, only to die there within hours or days. All of these patients had expected to die at home. How can we prevent this sort of thing from happening? — G.F., Pennsylvania

THE ABRUPT TRANSFER of a patient from home simply to die elsewhere a short time later rarely benefits anyone. So why does it happen? My experience with families who have a propensity to call 911 or show up at the ED has lead me to do two things: educate them better about what to expect and prepare them to handle problems. Here's how.

First, I discuss what family caregivers can expect at the end of life. In most patients, regardless of their illness, they can anticipate:

✦ lowered or undetectable pulse and blood pressure
✦ changes in level of consciousness
✦ periods of apnea.

When family members understand this, they aren't surprised when these signs and symptoms appear. I might reinforce my teaching by saying something like, "Remember, Ellen, we talked about how these breathing changes mean your dad is getting closer to crossing over?"

Second, I ask patients and caregivers what each of them fears most. Usually they say massive bleeding, choking, intractable pain, or confusion. Their fears may not all be realistic. For example, if the patient is dying of heart failure, massive bleeding isn't likely, and I can reassure them about this.

To allay fears, we can make preparations "just in case." For example, I keep a dark red blanket and towels tucked away for use during exsanguinations. (We all experience a primal reaction to the sight of blood flowing onto white linens.) Next, I go to the refrigerator, back behind the homemade noodle soup, and pull out the plastic box from the hospital pharmacy. The box contains emergency drugs for quick administration by the hospice nurse — injectable morphine, lorazepam (Ativan), and hyoscyamine sulfate (Levsin Drops) for that scary death rattle. I then discuss what each drug will do.

Finally, I have one more sit-down talk to remind everyone that the patient has an intense desire to die in his own home, amid familiar folks and surroundings. When nurses help caregivers believe they're perfectly capable of carrying out their loved one's wishes and do anticipatory problem solving, almost any hospice patient can die at home. ✎

Heart-to-heart talk

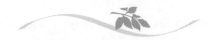

My husband has cancer of the bowel that has metastasized to his liver. I don't know how to tell our children — 7- and 9-year-old girls and a 4-year-old boy — that their father is dying. What would you suggest? — I.E., Pennsylvania

I'M TERRIBLY SORRY you're going through this. I can tell that deep down, you know it's time for a heart-to-heart talk.

Ask someone your husband likes and trusts to come and sit with him. Then take the children into one of their bedrooms, close the door, and pile onto the bed. Keep them close to you and to each other.

Some professionals would suggest that you talk to the children separately, but I disagree. I feel they should hear the bad news — as well as each other's questions — together. Besides, they're already feeling the tension and stress within the household. Taking one child away from the others to talk about something scary would only magnify their fears.

Allow at least an hour with them. Be gentle. You might start by saying, "I'm sure you know that Daddy is sick. He's much weaker than he was a few months ago. Sometimes doctors can't make people better. Daddy isn't going to get well."

They may ask you if their father is always going to be this sick. If so, they don't yet understand the seriousness of his condition. You'll have to tell them he's going to die.

Hug the children close to you and hold them tightly. Tell them you aren't sick and you aren't going to die, too. They need to feel safe, and they need to know that someone will take care of them.

You can remind your children that they can do special things for their daddy — for instance, taking juice to him or

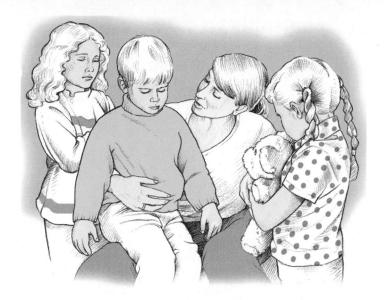

drawing him pictures. Including them in his care will help to reduce their fears.

You say the bowel cancer has metastasized to your husband's liver. I'm concerned about how his condition will change if toxins build up in his blood stream. For example, he may become jaundiced and confused—which obviously would frighten your children. You should prepare them by explaining that this change is part of his illness. Tell them that even if he doesn't seem to recognize them, he knows that his family loves him.

Encourage your children to ask questions, and give them brief, honest answers. Constantly remind them that you're still a family—and always will be. 🐟

Strangers in heaven?

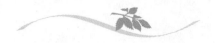

My 9-year-old son has recently expressed strong fears about dying. Part of his fear stems from the concern that he "won't know anyone in heaven." His father and I have tried to explain that he knows God, but his doesn't seem to satisfy him.

I'm puzzled by his sudden concern because all of our relatives and friends are alive and well. Any suggestions? — C.K., Ontario

I'M SURE YOU DID your best when you reminded your little guy that he "knows God." But I'm also not surprised that he wasn't satisfied— that response has failed to bring comfort to many adults.

Your son must be thinking that he'll die before you or his father. As a 9-year-old, he now understands death to be personal, universal, inevitable, and final. Scary stuff. No wonder he's afraid and asking questions. It's perfectly normal.

Talking more with him about your own religious philosophy might help. You can also say that, although it hasn't happened to you, you've heard about boys and girls who've come close to death and "crossed over," then returned to earth. These children describe beautiful gardens with trees, flowers, streams, and sunlight and many happy, loving people. They express a feeling of unbelievable peace. And they say they won't be afraid to die when their time comes.

These boys and girls also tell of their guardian angel being near, keeping them safe, knowing them all of their lives. (So, even though your son doesn't know his angel, his angel will know him.)

You might remind your son that even though he never met his great-grandparents or great-aunts and great-uncles, they'll recognize him and he'll be "greatly" loved and cared for.

At issue here, perhaps more than your son's feeling of isolation, is his fear of separation (innate to all God's creatures, I believe). He's growing up, and part of that growth is coming to realize that death is a part of life.

But only a part. So keep the focus on his schoolwork or his talents in sports or music, and let his day-to-day living take care of itself. 〜

What happened?

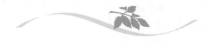

My manager's 10-year-old son was recently killed in a bicycle accident. She's just returned work. I feel bad about the pain she's suffering, but I don't know how to help. Do you have any suggestions? — C.H., Delaware

YES I DO — say, "I'm so terribly sorry about the death of your little boy. What happened?"

Then clamp an invisible hand over your mouth. In other words, keep quiet and just listen as she tells you the facts about the accident.

That's what I did after a favorite patient of mine died unexpectedly. It happened on a Saturday. When I returned to work the next Monday, the nurses filled me in on the details. A few days later, I saw the patient's girlfriend in the cafeteria. (She's a radiation technologist at the hospital where I work.) So I asked her how she was doing. When tears filled her eyes. I quickly guided her out of the cafeteria and into my office.

Although I knew most of the clinical details of the man's death. I asked her, "What happened?"

She began with his condition on Friday, after I'd visited to make sure he was comfortable. As her story unfolded, she began to cry, then sob. She continued talking, pausing briefly to wipe her eyes and blow her nose. I still remained silent, occasionally holding her hand or squeezing her arm reassuringly.

I gave her lots of time to tell me everything. That's one of the best ways to help a grieving person.

As difficult as it might be for you to sit patiently and listen to how your manager's son died, you'll help her more than you know.

Yes, it'll be tough. If you have children, you may feel guilty that they're alive and happy. You may also be anxious because the tragedy hit so close to home. And, certainly, you might be uncomfortable because this woman is your manager. Seeing her shaken and numb could be disconcerting.

Just try to see her as a fellow human being who's in pain.

Don't worry about saying the wrong thing to her. She'll remember only that you had the courage and sincerity to acknowledge her tragic loss and ask, "What happened?" ✎

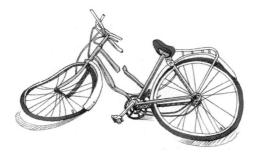

Keeping a secret

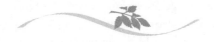

One of my patients has AIDS. He's told his wife, but he refuses to discuss his disease with his adult son and daughter. My nurse-manager and I think they have the right to know. How can we convince him to talk with his children? —R.D., *Nevada*

I DON'T THINK you want to manipulate a patient into doing something he doesn't want to do. That could destroy any trust he has in you.

I'm not sure why you think his children need to know. Because he's withholding the information, I assume your patient is ashamed about having the disease. (I'm sure just telling his wife was painful.) If he'd acquired HIV from a blood transfusion, he'd probably talk openly with his children. So my guess is that he acquired it from sexual contact or from sharing needles. Both modes of transmission are associated with behavior that society frowns on.

Perhaps you're interested in fostering honest, open communication among family members. I prefer that with my terminally ill patients, too.

But AIDS patients are different. Many people — health care professionals included — have the attitude that patients with AIDS "brought it on themselves." That kind of thinking changes the way some AIDS patients are treated. For instance, I've seen some of them badgered by health care professionals who want to know how they contracted the virus.

That's not the issue. What matters is that they be treated as any other patient would be — with the kindness and respect they deserve.

So don't focus on whether or not the patient tells his children that he has AIDS. Instead, concentrate on developing a trusting relationship with him. That alone is a challenge.

Also, explore the impact his disease has had on him and his wife. Try to move them through the guilt and anger they must be feeling—those emotions area waste of valuable time. As this process evolves, you might also talk with him about why he's so adamantly guarding his secret. And you might remind him that eventually, he should at least tell his children that he's dying. They may have some personal issues they need to resolve with him first.

Who knows? Once he feels accepted and supported, he may consider telling his children—not only that he's dying, but also that he's dying of AIDS. ✎

Plain talk

Last week, I accompanied a physician to our quiet room to tell a man that his father had died. Everything went well, but I was afraid the man would ask me questions that I couldn't answer. Do you ever worry about saying the wrong thing? —D.K., Ohio

I USUALLY FEEL comfortable in these situations. But a recent incident reminded me that I must always stay on my toes to avoid misunderstandings.

The ED staff paged me about a 76-year-old man who was being rushed in by ambulance. His wife had found him collapsed in the bathroom. The emergency medical technician had done an exemplary job of intubation and cardioversion in the field, but Mr. Rogers' heart wouldn't sustain a normal rhythm.

While the ED staff concentrated on Mr. Rogers, I sat with his wife of 50 years.

Excusing myself for a moment, I went to check on our patient. The ED physician reminded me to tell Mrs. Rogers that things didn't look good. (They'd attempted two more cardioversions.) I returned to her side.

"Mrs. Rogers, they're still working on your husband, but he can't hold a pulse."

She prayed; I held her hand.

When I checked again, the physician was gone and two nurses were clearing away equipment and supplies.

"We called it at 9:52," one of the nurses said. "Dr. Wright wants you to tell the wife."

I went back to Mrs. Rogers. In one minute, her social status had changed from wife to widow.

I knelt by her side and covered her hands with mine. "Mrs. Rogers, Mr. Rogers crossed over and decided to stay."

"Oh, thank you, Jesus!" she exclaimed and began kissing my hand. Horrified, I realized she'd misunderstood; she thought he'd survived.

I'd used those same words many times before without confusion. But Mrs. Rogers misunderstood because I'd talked with her about cardioversion and not being able to "hold" a pulse. No wonder she thought this last attempt resulted in his "crossing over" into a normal rhythm and "deciding to stay" in the normal rhythm.

The best advice I can offer is to speak the truth gently but plainly — using language the family won't misunderstand. ✎

Intrusive question

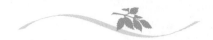

As a recent graduate, I read everything I can on death and dying. Last week, while administering a morphine dose to a woman with cancer, I followed your advice about communicating with patients and asked her, "How did you feel when the doctor said it might be time to stop the chemotherapy?" She appeared upset by my question and changed the subject. I thought I was supposed to ask patients how they feel. What did I do wrong?
—J.M., New York

YOU DIDN'T DO anything "wrong" in the context of being caring and concerned for her. But if you'll recall, my advice was to open the door to communication by asking, "Do you feel like talking about…?" Rather than demanding a response, this more subtle approach gives the patient a choice.

When you asked your patient to express how she felt—rather than asking if she wanted to talk about her feelings—you intruded on her privacy. No wonder she changed the subject.

Although you didn't intend to be coercive, consider her viewpoint: You're the caregiver who provides the morphine she needs. Because she depends on you, she may feel compelled to answer your questions, no matter how uncomfortable she feels.

Like many seriously ill patients, she'd probably appreciate a sensitive listener. But she might also feel that this whole cancer thing is too personal to discuss. If that's the case, she deserves to feel safe not talking and to know that this choice is perfectly acceptable too. ✎

Lighten our souls

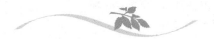

I'm a retired RN volunteering with a local hospice. I find I'm comfortable talking with my patients about death and dying. But is there a way to sometimes "lighten up" the conversation while remaining respectful? —R.C., *Missouri*

THE 17TH-CENTURY WRITER and moralist La Rochefoucauld said, "One cannot look steadily at either the sun or death."

It's perfectly right to provide relief from the seriousness of being terminally ill. But make sure you take your cue from the patient. If she's having an emotionally taxing or particularly painful day, it would be inappropriate to breeze into the room and fan out an array of photographs from your recent vacation. But it might be appropriate to remind her of her earlier interest in your trip and ask if she feels up to looking at photographs.

Most people appreciate the diversions. One way to offer a distraction from "looking at death" is to ask something like this: "If you were to wake up tomorrow all well, what would you do?" This question provides her with a wonderful opportunity to share the unfulfilled hopes and dreams of a lifetime. And it's especially meaningful to you to learn new things about the unique individual you're briefly companioning.

I was inspired by the courage of Martha, a beautiful lady terminally ill with leukemia, who agreed to be interviewed by me for a piece on "60 Minutes." At one point, we were discussing Martha's funeral. She wanted to ask her friend, the church organist, to play at the service.

"I'm not sure about asking her," she confessed.

"Oh, Martha, I think it's a lovely idea. I'm sure she'll be honored. Besides, you'd do it for her, wouldn't you?"

"Well, that would be hard," she replied.

Thinking Martha meant "emotionally difficult" I said, "But you'd want to be asked, wouldn't you?"

"I don't think she'd ask. I can't play the organ."

We both burst out laughing, as did Morley Safer, the producer, and the cameraman. What a precious memory for me. In the midst of this sensitive and reverent sharing, humor found its honest way to lighten our souls. ✍

2

Aiding the coping and grieving processes

Smoothing a rough road

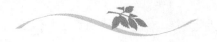

I'm fairly comfortable caring for dying patients. My problem is dealing with their survivors. Unlike you, I'm not a thanatologist. How can I comfort them in their grief? — *H.C., Illinois*

YOU DON'T NEED any formal preparation to help a grieving family. In fact, one of the most skilled "thanatologists" I ever met drove up to my farm on a front-end loader.

But let me start at the beginning.

I'd just been through a hectic week. I'd decided to practice what I preach and go play. So I went to the movies. Halfway through the show, thunder boomed. I was so absorbed in the movie that I hardly noticed.

Driving home, I saw a big rainbow. Things seemed right in my world.

As I entered the woods, I noticed that my lane was partially washed out; there were signs of flash flooding everywhere. But I'd encountered the worst.

When I approached my barn, I saw Cody, my wonderful little Morgan horse, lying dead in the pasture. He'd been struck by lightning.

I jumped out of my truck and ran through the wet grass. After examining him, I had to accept that my grand friend was gone. I sat with him for hours, then started to consider burial.

I called the man who'd done grading work on my driveway a few months before. As I started to speak, I began crying. Somehow, between sobs, he heard my need and simply said, "I'll see what we can do for you tomorrow morning."

A restless night finally turned into dawn. I went back to the pasture and paced in circles around Cody, like an Indian doing a dance of resurrection.

I heard the sound of machinery. Don drove the front-end loader into the field, then shut down the engine. I walked over to talk with him.

"I'd much rather dig up somebody's sewer line than come here to bury your horse," he said.

His sensitivity touched me, and I began crying again.

I picked a good spot, then did some chores while he dug. When he was done, he asked me if I wanted to go into the house while he dragged Cody's body into the grave.

"No, I'll stand by," I said. "He was a great friend. We played cowboys together."

I took my shovel—the same one I'd used 8 years before to dig my collie's grave—and gently covered the sleek, brown pony.

"You just take your time with that," Don said to me. "I'll take a walk in the woods if you want to be alone to say good-bye."

"No, but thanks anyway. I did last night," I replied.

He finished filling in Cody's grave, then gently smoothed the surface—an invitation for new grass to be planted.

I thanked him for his sensitivity. "I know how attached you can get to these animals," he said to me. "We've got two big German shepherds. They're our best friends."

He slowly drove away. Later, I walked out for the mail and discovered that Don had worked his magic with the front-end loader again. He'd somehow cleaned and repaired the flooded culvert.

He'd made the road a lot smoother.

And so can you, with kind words and sensitivity.

Symbols of solace

I was assigned to care for a terminally ill woman in our geriatric unit. Because she was aphasic from a stroke she'd had years ago, I had difficulty understanding her requests. One day, I'd almost given up trying to interpret what she was saying when her room-mate pointed to a seashell on the patient's bedside table. She'd realized that the patient wanted me to place the shell in her hand.

Once I did this, the woman settled down and fell asleep. She died peacefully that night. I'm not sure what therapeutic value that shell had, but it was obviously important to this patient. Have you ever heard of this kind of thing? — A.Y., Maine

YES; IT'S FAIRLY COMMON.

When working with terminally ill patients, we need to be sensitive to the emotional "healing power" of personal objects — which are often symbols of loved ones or happier times and places. As members of a materialistic society, we tend to be obsessed with accumulating "things." However, special trinkets can have spiritual value — providing solace to our souls. The memories we associate with these items may bring us more comfort than the actual presence of another person.

This was definitely true for one young man named Chris, who was dying of leukemia. He insisted on wearing a filthy New York Yankees baseball cap, which his estranged father had bought for him years ago on their only trip to Yankee Stadium. Although the father never visited during his son's illness and subsequent death, Chris always wore that cap — a tangible symbol of a distant memory.

I remember caring for Mr. Todorov, an elderly Russian whose wife Sophie had died in a concentration camp. To remember her, he always wore her locket around his neck.

Insights on death & dying

But his nurses were concerned that it would get lost or stolen, so they removed it and locked it in the narcotics cabinet. When he realized it was missing, he became frantic.

To prevent this from happening again, I put a sign over his bed, which read: DO NOT REMOVE LOCKET. Weeks later, when Mr. Todorov was near death, he motioned for me to come close. He opened the locket to reveal a faded picture of his beloved Sophie. Tears rolled down his face as he guided my hands to unfasten the clasp. He placed the locket in my hands, said a blessing over me, then lost consciousness.

I kept a vigil over him that night. And I kept the locket he'd entrusted to me. I know it will be one of the items I'll want to hold in my hand while I'm dying. I just hope there won't be any need for a sign over my bed. ✑

Say it with flowers

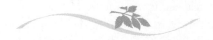

I'm writing on behalf of our pediatric nurses. Almost a year ago, a little girl named Amy died in our unit. I'd like to think that we love all our patients, but this child stole our hearts like no other. Most of the staff attended her funeral and have spoken by telephone with her mother. Do you think it would be appropriate for us to send flowers on the anniversary of her death? Our hearts say yes, but we don't want to upset Amy's mom. — *C.F., Arizona*

PLEASE ACCEPT my appreciation (and a big hug) to you and the other nurses for your compassion and caring. I believe we usually do better in life when we listen to our hearts rather than our heads.

Seven years ago, on December 23, the son of a close friend was killed in an automobile wreck. The boy, Ian, was only 19 years old, home from college for Christmas. His father, Keith, was the interior design specialist for my project for AIDS patients at York House Hospice, and I loved Keith for his commitment to me and my mission.

At Ian's funeral, the church overflowed with mourners. The family's home was flooded with flowers, cards, and visitors. Months later, things settled down and all the caring family members and friends went on with their lives.

When December 23 came the following year, I sent flowers and a note to Keith and his wife Nancy. And I continue to do so every December 23.

Nancy called recently to thank me. We talked about Ian and I asked if it was still a good experience for her and Keith to get the flowers.

"Oh yes," she said. "I always have to take the day off, and Keith always has to work." Now crying, she told me how meaningful the gesture is to them. "When I'm here at home thinking about Ian, I anticipate the delivery. Sure enough, it always arrives, and it's always beautiful.

"Joy, the biggest fear that parents have is that their dead child will be forgotten. Thank you so much for remembering."

And so, dear nurses, on behalf of Ian and Amy, I thank you too.

Gentle grief work

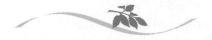

I recently began working in the ED of a large medical center, and I dread facing my first infant or toddler death. When this happens, what can I do to help the child's family? — *R.S., Quebec*

LET ME ANSWER you with a story.

One day, a young Chinese woman rushed to the hospital with her 7-month-old baby. He was dead, probably from sudden infant death syndrome.

Called to the ED, I found the woman rocking her baby. The thoughtful ED nurse had provided a rocking chair for her to sit in. Less thoughtful was the ED physician, who was peppering her with detailed questions about the cause of death.

"When did you find your baby?" he asked.

"At 6:30 this morning," she replied. "I was worried about missing my bus, so I...."

"When did you feed your baby?"

"About 7:30 last night. I gave him squash. Oh, my God! Did I feed him wrong? I feel like this is something I did wrong."

"Now those feelings don't do anybody any good," the physician said sharply. And he continued on with his questions, oblivious to her need for validation, clarification, and reassurance. He never touched the young woman or expressed condolences.

After he left, I took his seat and stroked the young woman's beautiful black hair. She kept saying, "Benny, you wake up now."

I asked if I could please see him. To my surprise, she handed the dead boy to me, saying, "Benny, Joy wants to see you. You be a good boy."

The blanket fell away, and I looked into his perfect little face. I told her he was beautiful and commented on his chubbiness.

"See, Jean, you did a wonderful job," I said. "He was [notice I used the past tense] healthy and strong. This was just a bad thing that happened."

I spent a half hour talking with Jean and her family — her brother and her father. (Her estranged husband couldn't be located.) When I asked her father if he'd like to hold his grandson, he nodded. Then he laid the baby on a stretcher and began to squeeze his tiny face and mouth in an attempt at resuscitation. When this failed, he rewrapped the dead boy and held him up, offering him to God.

Because the cause of death was unknown, the body had to be transported to the medical examiner, but the funeral director was unavailable for several hours. As time went on, I felt it was time to initiate some gentle grief work. I encouraged Jean to call her social worker and the child's godmother. She held the dead baby as she made the calls.

Often, nurses offer to make calls for the family. But the bereaved can actually take comfort from telling the story themselves.

I asked Jean if she'd like to place the ID bracelet on Benny's little leg. The same thoughtful nurse had made two so that the young mother could also wear one.

"Oh," she said, grasping his ankle. "He's so cold."

"Only his body is cold," I said. "The essence of Benny, his wonderful spirit, is perfectly fine."

I suggested she cut a lock of his hair. She loved the idea.

When the funeral director arrived, I prepared Jean and her family to let Benny go. "It's time to put Benny's dead body in the funeral director's car," I explained. "He put a little box in the back for him, and he promised he won't shut the lid." (I knew she'd have irrational — but still real — fears that Benny would suffocate.)

Handing the baby's blanket to the grandfather, I gave Jean a sheet to wrap her baby in. She smoothed his little shirt.

We walked outside to the funeral director's dark green vehicle. Its back doors stood open like wings; the little black box sat a few inches inside.

We all stood back and allowed Jean to tuck Benny in one last time. I was so proud of her. She'd come such a long way since 6:30 that morning.

Then she surprised me again by whispering, "Come alive, Benny, before it's too late."

But he didn't. So she asked him a second time.

Finally, she stepped back and stood between her brother and me...all of us crying in the bright September sunlight. ❧

Listen with your hospice heart

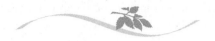

*I'm a hospice home health care nurse caring for a young man
named David who's dying of metastatic testicular cancer. His
parents are doing a fine job, but every day when his mother walks
me to my car, she asks how long this can go on. David is cachectic
and weak but still eats small meals. I don't know what to say to
her. What would you suggest?* — L.B., *Virginia*

FIRST, YOU MIGHT ponder why David's mother is asking the
question. It could be she's just exhausted. When she asks,
"How long can this go on?" she might really be saying, "How
long can *I* go on?" Or she could be asking because she doesn't
want to watch, one more day, her child dying. Possibly, it's a bit
of both. The important thing is that you "hear" her and provide
support without judging.

I can only imagine the agony this mother must feel as she
peeks into her son's room each morning to see if he's living or
dead. I wouldn't blame a parent for wanting the ordeal to be
over.

If David has been admitted to hospice, he probably has a
prognosis of weeks to months. Given your description of his
condition, that sounds accurate. David's mother may simply
need reassurance that her son's ordeal will end in the near future.

A horrific psychological factor for those imprisoned in Nazi
concentration camps was that they didn't know how long their
captivity would last, or if it would ever end. Most of us cope
better when we know that our turmoil has an end point.

Perhaps you can squeeze another hour into your next visit
to sit down and ask David's mother if she'd like to tell you
what these past months have been like for her. Encourage her

to share her feelings of lost hopes and dreams. You might also ask how she'd feel if David lingered for 3 or 4 more weeks. Could she get through that? If you listen with your "hospice heart," I think you'll find the best way to respond to her.

During your next team meeting, I also suggest that you make two requests. First, ask the hospice medical director to make a home visit. She's familiar with the trajectory of terminal illness and could provide David's mom with an educated guess as to how long David might live. Second, request more volunteer hours. If David's parents can get out for dinner or a movie, they'll receive a much-needed break—and a reminder that life still contains some normalcy.

Brooke's balloons

I'm the father of two toddlers, so when I care for a terminally ill child, I can't help but identify with the parents. I think about them for a long time after the child's death. How does anyone deal with such a heartbreaking loss? —M.M., New Jersey

EVERYONE COPES differently, of course, but some parents find comfort in keeping the child's spirit alive for themselves and others. Your question reminds me of Brooke, who died in the pediatric unit following a courageous battle with leukemia, and her parents, who were determined to memorialize her struggle. Members of her church collected money for a commemorative plaque, which her parents wanted to place on the door of the room where she'd fought her disease so bravely. But hospital administrators wouldn't allow it, afraid that many similar requests might follow.

The frustrated parents called me several times. Suddenly I had an idea!

I spoke with the child's pediatrician, who was also chief of the department. He agreed that something had to be done and made a few phone calls. The next day he proudly displayed the design of a large plaque to be placed in the hospital lobby. It would list the names of any children who'd died, if their parents chose to do so. Brooke's name would be listed first, with a few words describing how the memorial came to be created. It wasn't morose or scary, and hospital administration accepted the plan. Although Brooke's parents were pleased, they weren't completely satisfied. They still wanted her room to be special.

Suddenly I had another inspiration. Would they consider setting up a weekly delivery of nonlatex balloons to hang outside the door? They loved the idea.

"But what if a parent or child wants to know why the balloons are there?" asked the father.

"We'll just say because a very special angel wants them there to cheer up boys and girls who don't feel so good."

Brooke's father nodded, satisfied at last. "That sounds just like something our Brooke would say."

Grief takes a holiday

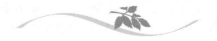

My next-door neighbors, a middle-aged couple and two teenagers, are lovely people. "You're a neighbor first and a nurse second" is how they describe me. So I guess the nurse in me is asking for your opinion.

The man's father, who'd lived with them for several years, died last month. A few days ago, the family left for Disney World. I'm doing my usual pet sitting for them, but I feel odd knowing these folks have taken their teenagers to have a fun time so soon after their grandpa's death. Am I being an old fuddy-duddy, or is this behavior acceptable in the name of grief? —N.M., Georgia

I THINK IT'S BEST to avoid judgments about how people handle a loved one's death. In fact, I'm probably quite alone in my belief that when it comes to grieving, no behavior should be labeled pathologic.

There's no book of rules. Mourning rites certainly differ among cultures, so why not among families and individuals? Wouldn't we expect coping mechanisms to vary among us, unique as we all are?

I'm reminded of a story about John F. Kennedy's family. After the death of his sister, his father, Joe, sat the brood down and informed them of the loss. Next, he announced that everyone was going sailing! Certainly, this isn't how most families would choose to cope with the sudden death of a young adult. But it was appropriate for this family.

You say your neighbors are lovely people and that Grandpa lived with them for a few years. Sounds good to me. Because we're not privy to their conversations, we don't know why they chose to make this trip. Perhaps they'd been planning it for years. Maybe on his deathbed, Grandpa made them promise to go, no matter what.

The point is that we don't know. It's personal. But we do know that they trust you to care for their pets. Maybe when they return, if they need to, they'll trust you with their hearts as well. ✎

Snapshots

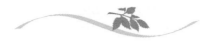

When my daughter had a stillborn baby, her nurse offered to photograph him. I know this is done at many hospitals, but these photographs make me uncomfortable. What do you think about this practice? — S.C., *Missouri*

I THINK IT'S HELPFUL. I understand your feelings, though: Many people are uncomfortable with a photograph of a still-born baby. But the loss is still the loss of a person, and family members must grieve.

The first task of grieving is to accept the loss. Photos help by showing the family exactly how the baby looked. They make the memory tangible.

In the past few years, more hospitals have been offering parents photographs like these. The baby is moved into natural-looking positions, and flowers, stuffed animals, and other toys may be used as props. Photographs with family members and friends of the parents can preserve the memory of all the supportive people who were present at the time of the death.

The response from parents has been positive. I've heard of some families who place the photographs in the family photo album. And why not? The baby was part of the family too. Trying to minimize the loss is wrong.

I suggest that you sit down with your daughter and look at the pictures together. Let her tell you about this special person and how she feels. Had she picked out a name? Does she worry that she'll never have a live birth? (Maybe you're wondering that yourself.)

She's hurting, and so are you. The best thing for both of you is to share your pain.

I'll bet the photographs help.

Mourning a classmate's death

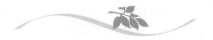

My brother's 7-year-old son, Mike, is grieving for a classmate who died about a month ago from a rare hematologic disorder. He's usually a tough little guy, but he sometimes breaks into tears when I babysit. Is this the kind of behavior you'd expect for a boy his age?
— *C.N., Virginia*

I THINK MIKE is expressing his grief normally. He may feel comfortable enough with you to release pent-up feelings that he's reluctant to express to his dad, precisely because he's always been labeled "tough."

As any pediatric nurse knows, children aren't just small adults, either physically or emotionally. They mourn differently than adults and have emotions they can't understand and worries they can't express.

Mike's crying is an expression of myriad emotions, one of which is anger. Like an adult, a child can get angry when he feels helpless and frightened.

Speak with your brother and ask if Mike is comfortable talking about his friend's death. He may be holding in a "secret." For example, he may feel guilty because he once told the boy he wished he were dead.

If Mike's intense mourning lasts more than 3 months or so, he may need professional counseling, especially if his emotions seem out of proportion to the loss or to his usual personality. Ask your brother about any red flags that might signal a need for intervention. For example, has Mike spoken about giving away his own possessions? Have his eating or sleeping habits changed? Does he seem preoccupied with death and dying or worried that he or others may die? Is he deliberately hurting himself? Has he lost interest in school? Does he have explosive rages and tantrums?

I think Mike's lucky to have you. The next time you're together, you might talk about how death is a part of life. Because Mike may worry that he'll die too, you could reassure him that it's rare for children to die. Remind him that he's a healthy boy and that you expect he'll be alive for many years. Also assure him that most people live to be old and that you don't anticipate dying, nor is it likely that his daddy will die soon.

You might encourage him to tell you about a happy experience he had with his friend. Then you can tell him that you're sure the boy was grateful that Mike was his friend and had fun with him. After all, that's what being a friend is all about.

Keeping memories alive

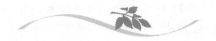

Five years ago, my friends were devastated when their 8-year-old son Doug was killed in a hit-and-run accident. They can't seem to let go of him: They've got pictures of him all over their home, his bedroom is virtually a shrine, and they hold a big celebration on his birthday.

They have two other children, so it's not as though they've been left childless. I'm beginning to think they've never really accepted their loss and are just prolonging their grief. Should I be concerned? — *F.T., New York*

I WOULDN'T BE — grief is a relative experience; there's no right or wrong way to do it.

I'm not disturbed by the birthday celebrations or the other sentimental gestures you mention. (Eliminating all signs of Doug *would* be upsetting, though.) These expressions of love set a nice tone for the whole family and provide Doug's siblings a chance to acknowledge and share their feelings about their brother.

I also don't think Doug's parents are consumed by grief. They seem to be dealing effectively with what counselors refer to as "shadow grief." Often associated with the loss of an infant or child, shadow grief is described as a cloud that's always in the background or a dull ache that never quite goes away.

Don't forget that Doug's death changed his parents' lives forever — nature doesn't intend for parents to bury their children. And having other children doesn't make up for their loss; no other child can possibly fill that special place in a parent's heart.

Doug's parents can't (and shouldn't have to) let go of their pain. It helps them hold on to their precious memories. ✍

Easing the pain

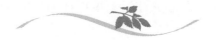

I'm a medical/surgical nurse. The patients on my unit aren't considered hospice patients, but they are terminally ill. I've noticed a commonality among most of them. Almost every one has a special object or picture that they bring to the hospital whenever they're admitted. Could you comment on this behavior?
—A.A., Rhode Island

GOOD FOR YOU for being so observant! When students make rounds with me, I always ask them to name three objects each patient surrounded himself with. My purpose isn't only to teach observational skills but also to remind them of the uniqueness and individuality of the "cancer of the bowel in Room 464."

I recall caring for a woman who had a nasty tumor of the jaw. Surgery had mutilated her more rapidly than cancer ever could, yet she retained a quiet dignity. With each hospitalization, she brought with her more malignancy and less flesh. But she also brought a photograph of herself on her wedding day—20 years before. She was a beauty. She wanted her doctors and nurses to see "who she was." Perhaps she worried that we would see her only as a distortion of the real her.

Special objects can also reinforce a patient's desire to extend his or her personality. A wonderful old cowboy was admitted to the hospital after being badly injured. He traveled with the rodeo and had no home or relatives. Aware of his impending death, he asked me to promise that he would die with his boots on. I did.

During my shift the boots stayed, but evening and night nurses removed them because they "dirtied the sheets." Three mornings I replaced the boots on his old, sore feet. Concerned that I had made a promise I might be unable to keep, I spoke firmly once more to the nurses, then posted a large sign over the cowboy's bed: "BOOTS MUST REMAIN ON PATIENT AT ALL TIMES."

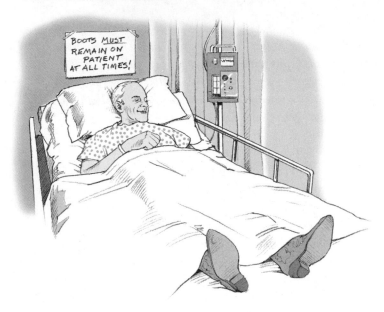

Finally, he seemed to trust that his wish would be carried out. He settled down and quietly died.

These special objects have meaning to family members as well. A daughter who arrived "too late" at her mother's deathbed took comfort in knowing she'd died with her head resting upon her daughter's embroidered pillowcase.

Some patients may want to drink "one more time" from a special cup or use real silverware to eat a bit of custard. You might want to place the meaningful object within the patient's sight, regardless of positioning. Flowers, too. Remember, the patient lying on his back sees only the ceiling or the overhead light.

You have good observational skills. I'm asking you to tap your imagination and help dying patients recall a few fond memories by providing them with a look at their living.

Put on a happy face

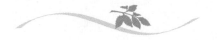

I'm a case manager in an inpatient oncology unit. One of our patients is a young man with bowel cancer and liver metastasis. We all know that he's dying. A few days ago he asked me to put a sign on his door saying, "Only smiling people may enter." I don't know what to think about this; it seems so false. What's your advice? — S.P., Ontario

A DEAR PATIENT once told me that he wasn't afraid to die until he saw fear in the faces of his nurses and doctors. Your moral, professional, and ethical responsibility is to take your cue from the patient. He's telling you loud and clear. "This is the way I need to do this right now."

He's not asking for everyone to be dishonest and pretend he's going to be cured. He's simply controlling the one thing left for him to control: the quality of his dwindling days.

I suggest you look for things about which you can be genuinely positive with this frightened man. For example, congratulate him on something he accomplished.

Once he feels confident that the staff will honor his request, he may move into a place of emotional safety and risk mentioning a fear or concern. Simply respond with, "I have some time now. Did you want to talk about that?" Don't be disappointed, though, if he chooses to remain silent and never discusses dying or death. Some people never do.

Remember, we invite the patient to dance, but we always allow him to lead.

Grieving doctor

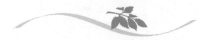

I was very surprised recently when one of our doctors began to cry as he was comforting family members at a patient's deathbed. He's not known as the emotional type; in fact, he's usually fairly cold and clinical. Have you ever seen this happen? —E.S., Wyoming

YES, I HAVE. A few weeks ago, I was at a luncheon meeting with my fellow clinical nurse specialists when my beeper went off. I was to go to the OR. I'm rarely called there, but when I am, it usually means the surgeon has found an unexpected, extensive malignancy.

As I went down the steps, I recalled some of my past experiences in the OR: comforting hysterical families, spending hours helping them process the bad news, preventing uncomfortable staff members from sedating upset and crying family members.

The surgical services nurse-manager took me aside and filled me in: A middle-aged man was having surgery to remove a large tumor on his kidney. Everything was progressing well—until his blood pressure suddenly dropped and his heart stopped. An aggressive resuscitation effort failed.

He just died.

Before seeing the family, I talked with the surgeon. He was devastated. His voice broke as he attempted to explain what happened. He mumbled something about giving up surgery. His eyes filled with tears when I put my hand on his shoulder. I had no words to take away his pain.

We went into the nurse-manager's office to see the patient's wife, daughter, and son-in-law. They, too, were devastated. The wife, now a widow, paced and sobbed. Her son-in-law held his wife close. The surgeon, who stood just inside the door, could only stare at his hands.

I arranged for the body to be washed and brought to a small room down the hall for viewing. The surgeon filed in with the family members. They sat in chairs that were arranged close to the side of the stretcher.

The patient's wife caressed her husband's face and hair, speaking softly to him as her tears fell on the green OR sheet. The surgeon leaned against the wall, staring at his feet.

I gently reminded the widow that she could stay for as long as she needed. She remained a few minutes longer, then said, "If I stay or go, it won't change anything." She was beginning to accept the reality of death.

Her son-in-law asked if they needed to sign any papers or do anything else before they left. I turned to the surgeon and asked if he'd requested an autopsy. He said he hadn't.

I rarely give my opinion to family members about an autopsy. But this time I did, for the doctor's sake.

I told the family that I thought knowing the cause of death would help their grief. "And I'm sure the doctor would like to know," I said. He could only nod in agreement.

A week later, the surgeon stopped me in the hall. According to the autopsy report, the patient had an undetected aneurysm that had ruptured. Nothing could have been done to save him.

Although the surgeon was still upset about the patient's death, he was able to walk through the swinging doors of the OR again.

Reserving judgment

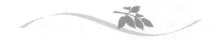

I'm a retired nurse, and I was glad to help care for a nice neighbor who was dying of cancer. His wife had died some years earlier.

His only daughter, who lived just an hour away, never came to visit him. But she did show up for the funeral, and she really made a scene with her hysterical crying — she even threw herself on him to kiss him good-bye.

She'd shown so little respect for her father while he was alive that this display was difficult to understand (and watch). Frankly, I was surprised that she attended. What do you think?
— H.P., Ontario

FIRST OF ALL, I think she had every right to be at her father's funeral, no matter how she behaved before he died. Funerals are neutral territory.

Second, you need to be careful about judging another person's behavior or intentions. A loved one's illness or death can bring out strange and confusing behavior. Neither of us knows why this man's daughter couldn't visit him while he was alive.

Remember, processing grief is very personal — there are no "shoulds." In other words, this woman wasn't doing what she *should* do; she was doing what she *could* to survive the wrenching experience of a loved one's terminal illness.

Finally, remember that you don't know enough about this woman's relationship with her father. You mention that he was "nice," but perhaps he wasn't that way with his daughter.

What's important is that you cared for your neighbor with a loving heart. Can you find compassion in that same heart for his daughter? I think your neighbor would want that. 🖎

Crossing over

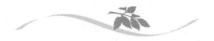

*I'm interested in why so many of us are afraid to die. If we really
believe what many of our religions teach us about heaven, why
don't we rejoice about "crossing over" to the afterlife?*
—*Y.L., Colorado*

THAT'S A GOOD QUESTION! Maybe because some religions
also teach about a punitive God, a hideous hell, and all sorts of
fearful images. That takes the naturalness out of dying darned
fast.

My experience with terminally ill patients has made me
think that our fear of death arises from our egos. Author
Deepak Chopra teaches us that the ego is our social mask. It
defines our role—who we think we are. Unfortunately, the
ego is fear-based and requires three things: control, power, and
approval.

Dying epitomizes the loss of control. Our body isn't the
servant it once was. It's unfaithful with its incontinence, its inability to perform familiar tasks, and its inconsistency in managing simple symptoms. Then comes the realization that our
physicians, with all their magic potions, are powerless to stop
this process. And we may not go gently into that good night.

The fear-driven ego constantly seeks approval. This is man-
ifested in the dying process by questions like this: "Why must
I die when I've been a good person and taken care of myself?"

The ego wants to deny the naturalness of dying, and it's
very serious about fooling us into thinking that we need control, power, and approval. But if we get the ego out of the way
and let in our true nature—love—then we can see that who
we are is more than the role the ego has us play. ✎

First patient death

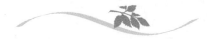

I know you've spent most of your career working in thanatology.
Do you recall your first patient death and what you were feeling?
—*H.G., Washington*

I WAS 17 YEARS OLD and had been a student at the Altoona
(Pa.) Hospital for about 3 months. Like the other new students, I hadn't been capped, but I was bursting with pride as I
strolled down that medical floor in my new starched uniform.

My first clinical assignment was an elderly man dying of re-
nal failure. He was barely conscious as I arranged linens and
toiletries for his bed bath. At first glance I thought he needed
a shave. On closer inspection, though, I realized his face was
covered with a salty, frostlike substance. Then I put together
his diagnosis and my assessment. He was being poisoned by
urea, which his failing kidneys couldn't excrete. It was escaping
like sweat through his pores.

Stopping in the doorway, my clinical instructor asked if I
needed help. I was about to say no, when the patient inhaled
deeply and never exhaled. I realized he'd just died. I looked up
for my instructor, but she was gone.

Not knowing what to do, I pulled the curtains around the
bed. I was about to go look for an RN when an on-rush of students led by a determined instructor entered the unit.

"Now you're about to see a case of uremic frost," I heard her
announce in her best tutorial tone. Before I could say a word,
she gave the curtains a firm yank and pulled them aside. I
stood uncertainly by the bed, a dry washcloth in my hand. Re-
alizing the patient had just died, the instructor quickly herded
my shocked schoolmates away without a word for me — or
him.

I had no idea if I should bathe the patient or wait for some special ceremony from his physician. Fortunately, one of the RNs came into the unit carrying a tray of medicine cups.

"Oh, honey. Are you okay?"

I nodded yes.

"I'll notify his physician. Just pull the curtains. I guess you should report to your instructor for another assignment."

I laid the washcloth on the bedside table and left. I felt sad and a bit embarrassed. In other circumstances the patient might have had a seasoned RN at his side, holding his hand and saying a few comforting words. Instead, he got a scared kid.

But I like to think that his death had meaning and that I was supposed to be present. Just maybe, his dying was the quiet inspiration that would lead me to so many other deathbeds in the future. ✍

Lost rituals

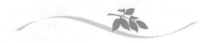

After my elderly aunt's funeral, we lingered at the grave site.
Something seemed to be missing. About a half hour later, we just
went our separate ways, still feeling incomplete. What happened?
— K.T., Kansas

I THINK YOU'VE just experienced the modern American funeral — not much substance, not enough ritual, and very little opportunity for participation.

Lingering at the grave was probably your attempt to experience a tangible closing. Unfortunately, the custom of lowering the casket in the presence of mourners has disappeared. The graveside service is usually brief, and most people simply return to their cars and their jobs. Their grief is probably complicated by the knowledge that they, too, will be buried with similar blandness.

This is not a fitting end to something as wondrous as the human body, a body that housed a soul.

Compare the American funeral with the customs of the island of Montserrat in the British West Indies.

The people there still observe the wake ritual. The deceased's family and friends gather on the night before the burial. They pray, tell stories, and eat and drink in his memory.

On the day of the burial, the body is placed in a simple coffin that has a window, so the mourners can see his face. Following the funeral service in the church, the body is taken to the cemetery, where selected friends of the family have dug the grave. Family members and friends toss dirt onto the coffin and in the grave, while all sing hymns that have been chosen by the family.

Everyone brings beautiful flowers, handpicked from their gardens. These are lovingly placed on the grave. No one departs until all of this has been done and family members have been greeted with hugs and kind words. This moving ritual means so much to those who participate.

I'm saddened that our few remaining funeral rituals are slowly disappearing. But I don't think this is entirely the funeral industry's fault. Consumers control supply and demand.

Grieving survivors have a right to insist on an individualized service.

I shout again and again that each of us is unique; none is like the other. Why don't we celebrate this uniqueness with specialized burial rites?

I love my little farm, and I want my coffin carried on a horse-drawn hay wagon. No shiny black hearse, because that's not me.

So if you have special and specific requests, speak up. In fact, it might make a great discussion at the dinner table.

Death of an iguana

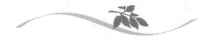

*I'm a pediatric nurse and the proud aunt of 10-year-old Brad.
Recently, Brad observed death first-hand when his dog had
puppies and all three pups died. Upset, he came to me because his
dad had told him he'd better not cry. I thought Brad needed some
understanding, so I told him he can cry with me when he feels sad.
What are your thoughts?* — S.D., *North Carolina*

I APPRECIATE your concern and I'm sure Brad does also. The
death of a pet is traumatic to most children and many adults.
But you're right. If handled with kindness and caring, the loss
can be easier to bear.

My friend Sharon shared with me the story of her 13-year-
old son, James, and the demise of his pet iguana, Dexter. It
seems the little lizard left the safety of his aquarium and was
attacked by the cat. After a tearful burial ceremony, Sharon
asked about removing the aquarium from James's room.

"I'm not ready to do that yet," he replied, and covered it
with a blanket.

Then James declared that he couldn't possibly attend school
the next day.

"I'll cry, Mom, and my buddies will make fun of me," he
said.

Sharon allowed him to stay home.

The next evening, Sharon found her son feeling less fragile.
He'd mourned and processed his feelings during his "grief
day," as we all must do. He greeted his mother with a hug and
asked her to help him move Dexter's aquarium to the garage.

You used your nursing instincts when you offered sincerity
and love to Brad. By not belittling his grief, you validated his
feelings. That's a good start to working through the pain. ✎

Hare-raising tale

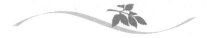

When our pet rabbit died, my husband took it to the veterinarian's office for disposal. Our 7-year-old daughter, Sarah, doesn't seem to understand what's happened. She says the rabbit has gone away but will be back soon. She spends hours near his cage, preparing his food and bedding. What should we do? —*M.P., Ohio*

GIVE SARAH LOTS of hugs and understanding, but don't get her another pet until she's accepted the rabbit's death.

I don't want to sound disrespectful or deny your daughter's pain, but the following story may lighten your load.

You may have even heard this story about a woman who found her large German shepherd sitting just outside the front door. A fluffy white rabbit was hanging limply from his massive jaws. The poor rabbit was bloody, muddy...and dead.

The woman recognized the bunny as the beloved pet of a little boy who lived two doors away. She felt terrible about what her dog had done. Quickly, she yanked him inside the house. After much praise for his hunting exploits and many thank-yous for his gift, she convinced him to give up his prize.

She bathed and scrubbed the dead rabbit. After blow-drying and brushing his fur, she stood back for a final inspection. Yes, he passed.

In the dark, she picked her way through the yards until she found the empty pen. As backyard noises echoed around her, she nervously placed the dead — but fluffy — rabbit in his cage, locked the door, and scurried back home.

The next morning, the boy's mother called to tell her that their pet rabbit had died — 2 days earlier.

And that they'd buried it.

"But now," she said excitedly, "I've found him all clean and pretty and back in his cage."

The woman was silent for a moment, then asked, "What are you going to do now?"

"Well, we'll have to bury him again, of course."

You can see the kind of trouble people get into by not dealing honestly with death.

Seven-year-olds certainly understand that death is final. But they also believe they can elude it if they're clever enough. Sarah may think your rabbit has gone away temporarily to fool death. She wants to make sure he has food and a soft bed when he returns.

I'd allow her to continue spending time near the cage, but I'd also gently remind her that the rabbit is dead and that the doctor buried it.

She probably would have benefited from some kind of funeral service and burial. That would have initiated questions about death and dying and would have been an excellent opportunity for you to chat with her.

Death is one of the most difficult lessons children have to learn.

But it's part of life, and with love and honesty, they handle it quite well.

Puppy love

As an ED nurse, I have a lot of professional experience with death and dying in the hospital. But when the pain hits home, I need help.

My 7-year-old son, Matt, is grieving terribly over the death of his puppy, who was hit by a car. I knew not to immediately replace the dog with another, but I did buy Matt a stuffed toy puppy. He's been lugging it around for 2 months, sleeps with it, and insists on taking it to school. Some of his classmates have been teasing him, but he seems to be okay.

A few days ago, his teacher called to tell me that she thinks this has been going on too long and that I need to stop Matt from taking the toy to school. Please help. My heart says it isn't hurting anyone, but my head tells me the teacher may be right.
—*J.K., New Mexico*

LISTEN TO YOUR HEART.

I think your idea was great. Too often, parents want to shield their children from the pain of loss and quickly replace the dead pet. Not only does this prevent the child from experiencing grief within the safety of home and family, but it may also make him believe that he too could be easily replaced, without a tear or aching heart.

The stuffed dog gives your little guy a sense of security and control. He's suffered a traumatic experience and is learning that life has some bad things in it. Snuggling a new dog that can never die is his way of regaining control over his world.

You and I do the same thing when we're in mourning. We might wear Grampa's old sweater or a favorite piece of jewelry from Aunt Irene.

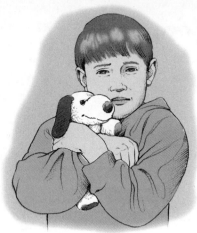

I like to remind people who have rules about grieving that we will grieve until we're done. For some, that may be weeks; for others, years.

Perhaps a telephone call to Matt's teacher would help. Simply explain that he's just a little boy with a sore heart. He'll leave his puppy at home when he's ready.

Gory details

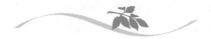

My husband Gary and I are both nurses — he works in the ICU of our local hospital and I'm an office nurse for a pediatrician. Gary is also an emergency medical technician (EMT). Although I'm proud of him for doing this, I'm sometimes repulsed by the gory, graphic details of his accident calls. But I feel guilty for not wanting to listen because I know he needs the support. What can I do? — B.K., Nebraska

YOUR HUSBAND'S NEED to relate these details isn't unusual — we all have it. When life's experiences are too overwhelming, we need to do something with the information. That usually means telling the story so that someone will acknowledge and validate events that have had a profound effect on us.

I certainly understand that you don't always want to hear the specifics. But I also know firsthand that humans can't help being affected by an accident.

Many years ago, I was the first to arrive at the scene of a two-car accident. It was dark, and the road was slick with rain. Two people had been thrown from one car; both were injured and unconscious. The driver of the other car, pinned upside down in his seat belt, was in shock. I quickly looked in what remained of the backseat of his car and saw the crumpled body of a woman. I felt around in the dark for her carotid pulse. Horrified, I discovered that she'd been decapitated.

I began shaking; my teeth chattered so badly that I thought my jaw would break.

By now, others had stopped to help. So I stumbled to my car and sat, paralyzed. I wanted to spare others this dreadful sight, but I couldn't get out of the car. About 10 minutes later, I quietly drove away.

Weeks went by before I could speak about this. Then, I had to tell everyone.

I suggest that you encourage your husband to talk with other EMTs or contact the county emergency medical services coordinator and ask to speak with a stress-management counselor. Or he can try talking with the ED staff—they're sure to be understanding, and may even have the same need to swap tales.

He might also consider keeping a journal in which he can express his feelings of rage and frustration as graphically as he wants.

Finally, remember that you don't have to listen to all of his stories, but you can still be there for him by making a special dinner, watching a funny video, taking a shower together, or just quietly holding him in your arms. ✍

"This is your life!"

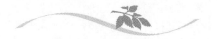

I recently read an article about a terminally ill man who decided to have a get-together for all of his family and friends so they could give him a proper send-off. The man was honored, teased and thanked for sharing his love, and it turned out to be a grand time for all.

I'd never heard of such a thing before, but I like the idea. Do you see any downside to something like this? — *C.D., Ohio*

I CAN'T IMAGINE that gathering all your loved ones together to give them an opportunity to tell you how much you've been loved and appreciated could possibly hurt anyone.

I initiated a similar "prefuneral" ceremony several years ago for a young high school principal who was dying from lung cancer. His staff asked me what they could do to honor his memory. They wanted to plant a tree or set up a scholarship fund. I thought both ideas were good, but I had another suggestion: Why not honor Kevin now, *before* he died?

Silence reigned for a few nervous minutes. Then suddenly they were all jumping out of their seats, eager to put together a "This Is Your Life" show for Kevin.

Given Kevin's state of health, I encouraged a speedy planning session that included an engraved invitation to Kevin. The gang put together one fine prefuneral party, and Kevin had a blast. His own two girls performed, as did kids from every grade level.

Kevin died a week later. I guess our timing was exactly right. ❧

Different reactions

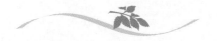

One of our obstetric patients had a miscarriage after 6 months. She seemed to handle the loss fairly well, but her husband was completely crushed by it. Do spouses usually grieve differently over a child's death? —R.F., Michigan

REGARDLESS OF SEX, all people grieve in their own way—but in general, men and women grieve differently. Men tend not to express their feelings as openly as women. Historically, they haven't had the "luxury" of grieving openly because their role was to provide the emotional (and financial) stability for the family. So their grieving was often delayed or suppressed.

To completely understand the reaction of this particular couple, I'd need more information; many variables affect bereavement. For example, was this her first pregnancy, or was it her third miscarriage? Was she ambivalent about the pregnancy? Do they have other children that she's especially concerned about right now?

Also, when you say she handled her loss "fairly well," do you mean that she cried a little or a lot? Perhaps she remained somewhat stoic precisely because her husband took the news so hard. It's very possible that *both* were completely "crushed" by this experience.

That's why you have to make sure that both parents participate in a grieving process immediately after the miscarriage. You can help to facilitate this by encouraging them to name their baby and, if appropriate, to bury him. This kind of ritual helps them to validate the miracle that their loving relationship created.

A touch of compassion

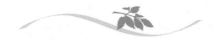

I'm the ED clinical coordinator. Last week, an 8-year-old girl was brought in dead from a motor vehicle accident. The child's parents were devastated and the nurses were at a loss to help them cope. Some of the nurses said they could barely get through it. What could we have done better? — *T.W., Tennessee*

IT SOUNDS AS IF this was an extremely difficult situation for everyone. The suggestions I offer come from years of experience learned, some days, by "barely getting through it" myself. Perhaps we need to be reminded that we're doing the best we can at all times and that we aren't perfect.

Let me begin by offering a few examples of what *not* to say to devastated parents:

+ "At least it was quick and she didn't suffer."
+ "You're lucky to have two other children."
+ "I guess God needed another angel to help in heaven."
+ "You can't fall apart; your family needs you."

These statements aren't helpful and belittle the parents' depth of loss. In contrast, the following statements offer compassion and support:

+ "I'm so terribly sorry."
+ "Would you like me to stay here with you, or would you prefer privacy?"
+ "I can't imagine how painful this must be."
+ "The old custom of saving a lock of hair has been helpful to people who are grieving. Would you like a lock of your little girl's hair?"

Grief work requires years of sorting out a gamut of feelings and emotions. But it begins at the moment the reality of death is faced. When that truth is grasped in a noisy, bustling ED, many nurses and physicians wish they had the "right words" to make the situation less horrific.

I'll tell you now, there are no such words. Nothing will blunt the pain of standing beside a dead child.

Years ago, at the end of a memorial service for families of dead patients, a mother said to me, "I don't remember any of your words as you sat with us over Steven's broken body. But I'll never forget when you took my hands in yours and just shook your head in sorrow. You even had tears in your eyes. Somehow, you almost understood our grief at that moment."

I don't have any profound wisdom to give you or your staff, except to remember the humanness that we all share. Don't try to find the perfect words. Just let your genuineness speak for you.

Making decisions

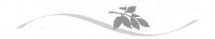

I'm a 29-year-old medical/surgical nurse. Six months ago, my husband died on the ICU of the hospital where I work. Since then, I haven't been able to get over the emotional strain. To make matters worse, my manager seems to expect me to behave as if nothing has happened. I'm considering leaving this job. What do you think I should do? —D.F., California

I'M NOT QUALIFIED to advise you about taking a specific action; nor would I be comfortable doing so. But I can share my thoughts about what might be happening with you.

First, you needn't be concerned that you're still upset and depressed. Six months isn't enough time for you to have finished grieving. I strongly believe that you need to go through this time of healing at a pace that feels right for you.

There are no "shoulds."

As you point out, you have choices. One of them is to leave. But don't be fooled into thinking your grief won't follow you. You'll still be going through the grief process. And you might feel a second loss when you leave co-workers you've become especially close to.

Maybe you prefer a change of scenery, but that can be stressful even if the move is good. So I suggest that you sit down and make two lists: one of the good and bad points of remaining, and the other of the good and bad points of resigning. Be honest with yourself.

If you decide to stay, you might want to meet with your manager and share your feeling about what you perceive to be her nonsupportive behavior.

Here's a point to remember when you're talking with her: A death can affect others in unexpected ways. Your manager, for instance, might be feeling guilty because her husband is alive and well.

Ask her for feedback about your nursing care. Does she think it's been compromised by your emotional stress? If so, you might consider taking a break from hands-on, bedside care. Your patients need competent, considerate care. There's no disgrace in stepping back and taking time to regroup.

Many health care professionals are reluctant to admit that they need help. But you do. Ask your social services department for information about a local support group for widows, preferably one that includes women close to your age. They can be of great help.

There are no wrong decisions.

Your difficult days will become fewer. You'll heal and smile again. ✑

Sense of humor

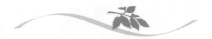

My uncle died last week. I loved him and always enjoyed his wonderful ability to laugh at life. As we were driving to the cemetery, the hearse carrying Uncle Jack had a fender bender with a meat truck. I thought it was funny and started to laugh. My sister, who was in the car with me, told me I was sick. What do you think? —F.B., Pennsylvania

IT *WAS* FUNNY. And I'll bet Uncle Jack giggled right along with you. Actually, laughter is great for relieving the tension surrounding death and bereavement.

I remember many funny moments from funerals I've attended. Once, a funeral director thought he knew where the entrance to the city's largest cemetery was located. But as he drove up, he realized he didn't. So he was forced to drive around the outside of the cemetery again.

Convinced the gate was on the north side, he continued driving, with a lengthy procession following. Again, he missed it. Finally, on the third time around, he found it.

At the graveside, the widow whispered to the driver of the hearse that it was terribly thoughtful of him to "drive Henry around the town for one last look."

Here's another one, told by a minister. Rain was coming down hard the day of the service, as it had been for several days. The family was seated on folding chairs inside the tent.

The deceased was a retired military man. At the moment of the 21-gun salute, the widow's chair collapsed, dropping her into the mud. Her 8-year-old grandson jumped up and shouted, "Oh, no! They've shot Grandma!"

So, I don't think there's anything wrong with finding humor in grave situations (pun intended).

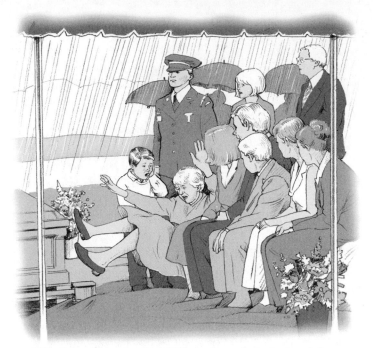

We all express our grief differently — there isn't a right or wrong way to do it.

Hats off to you for loving Uncle Jack when he was alive and for allowing his sense of humor to help you through your loss.

Look to the past

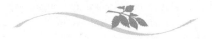

One of my patients is dying of liver cancer. He's a warm, funny man — even when he's in pain — and I enjoy talking with him about his family and hobbies.

One thing bothers me though: Whenever his wife or daughter mentions his illness, he makes a joke and changes the subject. Should I be concerned that he isn't facing his death?
—E.M., Kansas

HE IS FACING his death, in his own way. We're all fairly predictable in the way we cope with crises. Your patient has probably laughed off past disasters to protect his family from pain.

The next time you have a quiet moment alone with him, I suggest you ask him how he got through other painful times in his life. As he recalls the way he handled past crises, he may find another way to deal with this one.

That's what happened with Arthur, who didn't want his wife, Mary, to know he was dying. "I don't know if you've met her," he told me, "but she's just a little thing. I don't think she could take this kind of news."

I asked Arthur what troubles he and Mary had shared in the past. "Well, we had a stillborn baby," he said, his eyes filling with tears. "I guess we just held on to each other and talked it through."

"Yes, and don't you think holding on to each other and talking is the best thing to do now?" I asked. "I'm afraid this is the worst crisis you and your wife are ever going to share."

"Yeah, you are right," he said finally. "Say, would you come around later, when she comes in to visit?"

"You bet."

Ironically, I didn't have to wait. I ran into Mary in the coffee shop and we sat down to talk. When I asked her how sick her husband was, she looked down and shook her head.

"Oh, dear," she whispered, "he's dying."

"Yes, I know. He told me today."

"*He* told you?" she asked, not believing me.

"Yes, but he felt he needed to keep it from you."

She shook her head. "I've known all along. I asked the doctor not to tell him, though, because I just didn't think he could take it."

"He said the same thing about you. After talking with both of you, I think it's time to bring this out in the open. How would you feel about that?"

She started to cry. "Well, I'm a little afraid. But you know, dear, I surely do love him."

"That sounds good enough to get you two through this. Come on, he's waiting."

After seating Mary in a comfortable chair at her husband's bedside, I pulled the heavy, yellow curtain around them. I promised to return in an hour.

When I did, I found Mary leaning her head on Arthur's pillow. Both of them were weeping as they discussed who would get Arthur's gun cabinet and truck and when they should bring their son home from Colorado. The whole cloud of pretense had disappeared as they prepared to face death as they'd faced life — together. ✑

The little matchmaker

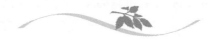

My husband died 4 months ago at age 38. Over the last 6 weeks or so, our teenage daughter has become obsessed with the idea that I should remarry. She waits up for me when I go to a party to find out if I've met a prospective husband, and she's even asked some of the male teachers at her junior high school if they're available. I'm very concerned about her behavior. What can I do?
— N.H., Illinois

FIRST, TAKE YOUR daughter's hope that you'll remarry soon as a compliment. She obviously saw your relationship with your husband as happy and positive. And she wants you to have a new husband so you'll be happy again.

Her desire to have a father also speaks well of your husband. He must have been a good dad.

You don't mention how you're coping with your husband's death, but I'm sure you're going through some tough times. For the moment, though, you may have put your own grieving aside to focus on your daughter's matchmaking efforts. Just remember that her intentions are pure: She may hope that having a new husband will make your pain — and hers — simply vanish.

Unfortunately, you and I both know that it won't.

She needs to experience sad feelings for quite a long time. Then, when they begin to go away, they'll stay away for longer periods. If she tries to push away the pain, she may find that it's even stronger when it returns.

So, what can you do? Start by having a heart-to-heart talk with her. Perhaps you could plan a picnic lunch on her bed (her turf). Tell her that you want to talk about your feelings, and ask her if she wants to talk about hers. This will let her know that you're feeling pain over your loss and that you want to share it with her.

Remind her (and yourself) that crying is okay. You've both experienced a terrible tragedy. Acknowledging it may lessen the pain.

Explain to your daughter that you're still a family — even if just two of you are left. And let her know that although she's growing up in many ways, she's allowed to feel like a little girl when she's frightened or sad.

Now more than ever you need to set aside a little time to talk with her after school. Just sit and chat about her day for a few minutes. You might even gently tease her about looking for husband/father material at school. The important thing is for her to feel comfortable expressing herself and to see that you do too.

This pain and sadness that you're now experiencing will eventually subside, and you'll both begin to feel happy again. One of these days, a special someone will come into your lives. Until then, you can lean on each other. ✎

Doing the dirty work

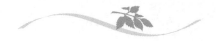

Several weeks ago, the husband of a nurse I work with died in a skiing accident. The entire staff was terribly shaken, and we didn't know what to do for each other. It helped that we attended his funeral, but now, weeks later, we're still upset. Is it too late for us to find some kind of support? — *T.S., New Hampshire*

NOT TOO LATE at all. Grief has a way of staying with us, so I suggest you seek a kind of ongoing support that acknowledges each person's approach to and pace of processing the grief.

My team members and I suffered this same anguish when a staff member's son was killed in a car crash. We all were in shock, with many nurses crying openly as they tried to care for patients. I sought out a dear friend in another department because I quickly realized that I needed to be consoled before I could console others. At that moment, I had little to give.

So I did what I advise others to do: I was honest about my own pain. It seemed as if sharing it with others who were also horrified leveled the playing field. I might have read the books and attended the seminars, but this time I was among the forlorn. My teammates and I then engaged in an ancient ritual: gathering together, holding each other, and crying.

You too must acknowledge your loss with others because you'll all be affected for quite some time. Remember, even when we share the same loss, we cope differently, according to our own history. It'll help if you meet and "tell your stories" so that each of you receives validation of what this particular death means to you.

Grief is dirty work, and we don't like doing it. But as I must remind myself at times, it must be dealt with eventually. Face it head-on now so it doesn't haunt you in the future. ✎

Burial gifts

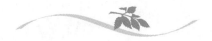

My neighbor was killed in a farming accident a few weeks ago. Because I babysit for his grandchildren (ages 6, 8, and 9), I offered to accompany them to the funeral. When I picked them up, the children were toting items they wanted to place in the casket — an old baseball, a shaft of wheat, and a Spiderman comic book. What do you make of this? — M.M., Kansas

RECENTLY, I DID a bereavement follow-up with a young mother whose 4-year-old had been killed in a freak accident. She told me how she and her two other children placed various items in the small coffin — several of his favorite toys, candy, books, and a Power Ranger belt. She asked if I thought she was crazy, and I replied, "Absolutely not."

This burial custom is ancient — and nearly universal.

We're all familiar with the discovery of King Tutankhamen's tomb in Egypt some years ago. While visiting the Cairo museum, I toured the collection of the royal treasure. Included were the boy king's favorite toys, foods, games, and weapons. Outside the entrance to the burial chamber stood two wooden guards the exact height of Tut — provided, like Power Rangers and Spiderman, for protection.

Tut died nearly 3,500 years ago. Yet we know of graves 70,000 years old that also contain items intended for use in the afterlife.

So no, I don't find the gestures by your friend's grandkids peculiar. I think these children are just responding to an ancient memory. 〜

3

Handling sensitive family issues

The parent trap

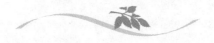

I'm having trouble accepting my mother's dying process. We're fairly close, but we've never been like some mothers and daughters who are best friends and do everything together. Mom was a pillar of the family. She took care of us and always seemed capable and in charge. Now I have to bathe her, feed her, and do just about everything else for her. My father tries to help, but both he and my mom expect me to just take over. I think I'm doing okay, but I do feel somewhat confused and frightened. What's wrong with me?
— *L.K., Rhode Island*

I DON'T THINK anything is wrong with you.

You and your parents have reversed roles, with you becoming a sort of parent to them. They raised you, nurtured you, and protected you. Now you're doing for them many of the things they once did for you — with one major difference. You haven't chosen this role.

I can see why you're feeling confused and frightened. As a nurse and a daughter, you feel obligated to care for your parents, and you don't have the luxury of collapsing under the weight of grief and impending loss. And your mom is abandoning you. Even though you're a grown woman, fully capable of working and making a place for yourself in society, you're also a little girl, used to Mom always being there. Your response to all this is normal.

Another difference in this situation is the fact that every day, week, and month of your childhood, you were growing more independent. With your mother now, it's just the opposite. As she becomes more dependent, your commitment to her care can only become more involved…with more sleepless nights, more days of feeding, bathing, and giving—all while you're preparing yourself emotionally for a huge loss.

I suggest you consider getting some friends, siblings, or neighbors to lend a helping hand. Believe me, no one does this alone. And it simply isn't fair for anyone—even parents—to "should" all over someone else.

Years ago, I worked with a nurse who promised her dying father that she'd always take care of her mother. A few years later, the widow developed numerous ailments and insisted her daughter move in with her. My friend complied.

Then, after more illness, surgery, and dependency, the mother demanded that the daughter stop working and care for her full time. Again, she complied.

But in a strange twist of fate, my friend developed a life-threatening heart condition that began draining her strength. During a visit, I reminded her that she could still keep her promise by using different ways to "take care" of her mother. For example, she could admit her mother into an extended-care facility or insist that her eight siblings help with caregiving or pool resources to get live-in help.

She chose none of the above. Instead, she chose to die of a heart attack. Now the mother's in a nursing home, and the other children don't visit much.

Please make some calls today. You don't have to lose yourself as well as your mother.

Choose to let go

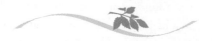

My mother recently had my father admitted to a nursing home. He has Alzheimer's disease, and she says she can't care for him at home anymore. I'd like to pitch in, but I'm working full-time and going to school to get my BSN. Dad always said he didn't want to end up in a nursing home. Now I'm so angry with my mother that I haven't spoken to her in weeks. How can I get her to change her mind and bring Dad home? — M.P., Arkansas

YOU CAN'T. And you'll never find peace if you hold on to your anger.

I'm sure this was a difficult decision for your mother. But she was honest with herself — she doesn't think she can be your father's primary caregiver.

That's fine. She made a choice and she's following through with it.

You also have choices. You could have your father transferred to your home and hire nurses to care for him around the clock. That can be expensive though, which may be why your mother didn't choose it.

Or you can accept that all things are happening exactly as they're supposed to, even though you don't like the situation.

Also, you can choose to forgive your mother — it's what you both need. This time is difficult enough. You don't need the added stress of tension, anger, and resentment.

Your mother is doing the best she can. And so are you.

Choose to let go — choose peace over conflict — then watch what happens. Your mother will feel more comfortable. Your visits with your father will be much more pleasant. (He'll sense your peacefulness.) Then you can all take loving care of each other. ✎

Soldier in arms

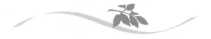

My patient has two teenage daughters. Her malignancy is out of control, but she keeps asking the physician to do everything to keep her alive. I think she and her family need to talk about her condition and prepare for her death. —*J.N., Alberta*

DON'T ASSUME you know what she's told her family. She may very well have talked with them about her illness but is choosing to say, "I have cancer, yes, but I'm not going down without a fight." I suspect she feels that every day she spends with her young daughters is precious.

I was honored to work with a young wife and mother who was devoted to her 11-year-old daughter. She'd been "battling" (her word) breast cancer for 7 years. Metastases to the lung had triggered recurring pleural effusions. Repeated thoracentesis offered only a few days' relief from terrifying sensations of breathlessness.

I'd known her only a few days when we sat quietly watching her favorite talk show. Gently, I broached the subject of hospice by asking if things were getting too difficult these days. She smiled weakly and nodded yes. Certain that she'd welcome the chance to stop futile treatments, I innocently asked, "Do you sometimes feel like giving up?"

She pushed herself to a sitting position and said defiantly, "Absolutely not!" I knew she was thinking about her daughter.

I reminded her of my commitment to her and her family and said I'd be an advocate for her in every aspect of her illness.

Be your patient's nurse — even her confidant. But most important, if she chooses to fight on, be her soldier in arms. 〰

Youngest pallbearer

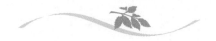

My mother-in-law, who's lived with us since my daughter Michelle was born, is dying. Michelle, age 9, adores her grandmother and will miss her terribly. When my husband and I talked to Michelle about the funeral, she asked to be a pallbearer. My husband said, "Absolutely not!" Michelle asks again every day, even though my husband has explained that only men can be pallbearers. What are your thoughts? —E.F., Ohio

I THINK YOUR daughter would make a fine pallbearer. Customarily, men perform this role because of the casket's weight. But I've seen women and children participate in this ritual too.

Pallbearers typically are close relatives or friends of the deceased or his family. Next of kin are commonly excused in deference to their grief, although some sons insist on helping to bear the body. Being asked to serve as a pallbearer is an honor.

I'll never forget the funeral for a young girl who'd died in a car crash. Several gentlemen acted as pallbearers, but one of the girl's classmates walked alongside them, her hand touching the casket.

So I see no reason to deny Michelle's request. She doesn't need to be physically capable of bearing the weight; just squeeze her in next to one of the men, perhaps her dad. She may want to participate in the funeral in other ways too; for example, by giving a tribute to her grandmother during the service. Allowing her to participate in the service and express her grief in a visible and physical way will help heal her heart. ✎

Eye on the sparrow

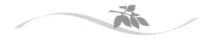

I work in a progressive care unit in a rural area. I'm often involved with families of dying patients. In their grief, they're usually anxious and they can't settle quietly at their loved one's bedside. How can I help them? — *P.M., British Columbia*

LET ME BEGIN with a true story about Elyse, whose mother was going through a hard death from lupus. Hospitalized for over 2 weeks, the patient was struggling to breathe, even on 100% oxygen. Totally exhausted, Elyse left the hospital to go home for a rest. She remembers crying to God, asking why her mother had to suffer so.

Falling asleep, she dreamed of a tall, lit candle. Flying near and around the candle was a small brown bird. At one point, the bird flew too close and the flame set fire to its breast feathers. Elyse began throwing water on the bird, trying to extinguish the fire. *Little birds shouldn't have this happen to them*, she thought. *This shouldn't happen.*

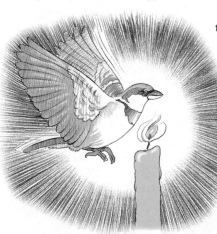

While driving back to the hospital, Elyse recalled that her mother's favorite hymn was "His Eye Is on the Sparrow." This triggered her memory of the dream. Rerunning it in her mind, she suddenly understood her dream's message: She was trying to stop something in nature that was unstoppable. Finally at peace, she found a renewed energy and purpose in the last few days of her mother's life.

You might find it helpful to gently share this story, then ask your patient's family and friends if they can recall their own dreams. Even if the message isn't as obvious as the one Elyse described, expressing these subconscious thoughts can help families explore their fears about the physical changes in the dying person. (Of course, do this away from the bedside.) Allay their fears by explaining how the care team will help manage the patient's pain. Tell those keeping watch about the changes in rhythm and depth of breathing. And speak as if the dying person can hear and is just too weak to respond.

Stay near and check in frequently, without being intrusive. Remember, this isn't your family. It's their time. Soon enough, you'll be in their place.

Cat controversy

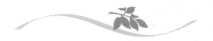

A woman I'm caring for has come to terms with the fact that she's dying of congestive heart failure. The problem now is her cat Tiger: She says she wants him put to sleep when she dies because she doesn't trust her husband to take care of him. The husband, though, wants to keep the cat as a sweet memory of his wife. My patient becomes very agitated whenever they discuss this. How can I help them resolve the situation? — D.G., Minnesota

WELL, I SUPPOSE the most obvious solution is for the husband to agree to her request, then not go through with it. But I doubt that he'd feel good about lying. And he may have trouble with the grieving process later if he feels guilty that he deceived his wife and didn't honor her request.

I think you have to look at what else is going on here. Your patient says she can't trust her husband to take care of Tiger. Maybe what she's really saying is that he doesn't take good care of *her*. So she's getting back at him the only way she can — by denying him a chance to care for the cat.

That's not unusual. I've known some dying patients who were so bitter that they tried to punish their spouses. If your patient deeply resents her husband, she may not want him to take any comfort from having the cat around after her death.

You may find that the cat is a symbol of control for her — and she's definitely in a situation that's otherwise beyond her control. So talk with her about *why* she wants to have Tiger put down after her death. Bring up the issue of trust. What does she think would happen to the cat if her husband kept him? Does she worry that her husband would neglect or mistreat him?

This dispute over the cat could be a symptom of a larger problem. Try talking with your patient and her husband. Help them explore their feelings about their life together and her imminent death. The three of you should be able to find a solution that will put your patient's mind at ease and give her husband the comfort he wants. ✎

Coping with fear

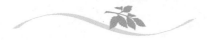

I'm an RN in a large oncology unit. One of our patients, who's been admitted numerous times before, probably won't survive his current admission. The strange thing is that his wife, usually so open and realistic, suddenly refuses to let us discuss death or dying with her husband. How should we handle this? — *E.S., Colorado*

THIS REACTION could be a normal coping mechanism for her. During a long terminal illness, patients and family convince themselves that living with cancer isn't so bad because at least they're still together. But as the possibility of loss looms closer, reality gets pushed aside to try to stave off the inevitable.

I'm not saying that denial is necessarily a bad thing. By serving as a buffer, it can allow people time to absorb bad news so they can process their feelings.

In trying to protect her husband, your patient's wife may really be trying to protect herself. Maybe she's never held a job outside the home and has no marketable skills or experience dealing with household finances. Perhaps she doesn't drive. Any one of these problems, let alone the terrifying thought of her husband's death, is enough to cause her anxiety.

You might sit with her privately and ask what losing her partner means to her. She may be reluctant to share her inner feelings because she believes it would be selfish (family members often say they aren't entitled to feel sorry for themselves).

You'll need to use your communication skills to help her share all her fears. Be sure to remind her that she's stronger than she thinks. And ask her to remember how she survived crises in the past.

If you feel uncomfortable in this role, ask a psychiatric clinical nurse specialist, hospital chaplain, or grief counselor to talk with her. ✎

Who's keeping watch?

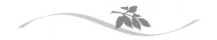

In our oncology unit, several patients die each week. Recently, a patient's adult son refused to stay with his father, even though we explained that death was imminent. I think the son should have stayed. It was his father, for goodness' sake! What do you think?
—E.H., Vermont

I THINK WE have to be careful not to "should" all over each other. Your opinion about this son needing to stay is just that—your opinion.

You did well to offer information about the patient's impending death. The point is, he *chose* not to remain. We don't know why—nor do we need to.

I recall working with a sweet gentleman who'd been slowly dying for several days. His lovely wife had been keeping watch the entire time...eating and sleeping in his room. Suddenly, she announced that she was going home and asked that I call her "when it's over." Stammering with amazement, I agreed.

She must have sensed my surprise, because she explained that she and her husband had agreed that he'd die without her being present. She smiled at me as the elevator doors closed. A few hours later, as promised, I called to inform her of her husband's death.

I believe the lesson here is that even though many individuals choose to remain at their loved one's deathbed, some choose to leave. And that decision has nothing to do with you or me. They are each individuals, and each death is unique. Our concern is to ensure that our dying patients have a dignified passing, regardless of who's "keeping watch." ❧

A little understanding

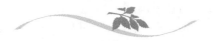

My 36-year-old brother-in-law is dying of liver cancer. As if that weren't enough, my nephew, who's 15, has been acting up; in fact, he was just arrested for stealing a car. I know this behavior is breaking my sister's heart. How can we make him understand what's going on? — K.S., Connecticut

HE DOES UNDERSTAND. That's the problem.

I'm sure that if you asked him, he'd tell you that he only wants you and his mother to understand what he's going through. After all, he's losing his father.

I can't imagine what a tough time this must be for him. But I do recall how difficult 15 can be — trying to test the waters of independence without giving up the security of home…feeling invincible one week, homely and insecure the next…constantly hearing the "don'ts," as in "Don't stay out after 10" and "Don't use that kind of language."

On top of that, your nephew is getting other restrictions:

✦ "Don't play your music too loudly. It bothers Dad."

✦ "No, I don't think you should go to the concert."

✦ "Don't bring your friends here after school. You know your father is sick."

So now what you have is a young man who really needs to go fishing with his dad and talk about school and girls and life and…everything.

But his dad can't do that, and a lot of anger and energy are building up. So he acts out.

As I see it, right now he needs to hear some "do's" like these:

✦ "Do you want to talk about what losing your dad is like for you?"

✦ "Do you want some time alone with Dad?"

✦ "Do you think you could help Dad shave?"

Stealing the car was a symbolic act. Your nephew was trying to get away from the scary world he's in. He may feel an unspoken expectation that he'll be the "man of the house" now. And that just may be too much for him.

If possible, you or a close family friend might make time to take your nephew to a ball game or the movies. It really doesn't matter where you go. He just needs to feel that someone — an adult — is there for him. I'll bet one of his biggest worries is that no one will take care of him, although I doubt he'd want to admit it.

I think your nephew is crying for help in a language that's acceptable for a 15-year-old boy who's watching his father die. He's asking, "What about me?" — a perfectly normal concern. (We all ask it, just in different ways.)

So try to cut down on the "don'ts." But add a more valuable one: "Don't forget that we love you." ✍

Greetings for the future

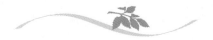

My sister Lois has ovarian cancer and will probably die before Christmas. My heart is breaking for her 17-year-old daughter, Jenny, who's devastated by this tragedy. Lois wants to sign a graduation card for Jenny now, then have me give it to Jenny next spring. I feel okay about this, but what's your opinion?
—*I.W., Quebec*

I THINK it's a wonderful idea. I know of another family that did the same thing. The young mother, also dying of cancer, bought numerous cards for various occasions and wrote a little note in each. Over the next 2 years, the father gave his daughter these precious cards for her birthday, Christmas, and her high school graduation.

I like it. I don't believe it's pretense, denial, or anything other than a special kind of loving. The dying mother did indeed send these well wishes. She just postdated them. ✎

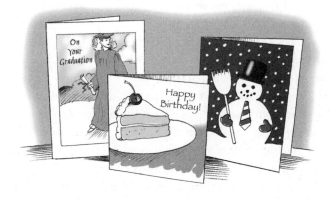

Memento mori

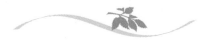

As a nursing shift coordinator, I feel comfortable with most death and dying issues. So asking for advice is new for me.

My dad died several months ago; his body was cremated. Last week when I visited my mother, she showed me the urn containing Dad's ashes. She has it on the mantel above the fireplace, like a souvenir from some trip they'd taken! I'm distressed by this but wonder if I'm overreacting. What do you think? —B.H., Illinois

I'D LIKE TO remind you that feelings aren't right or wrong. They're just feelings. It's perfectly natural to be confused when you're bereaved.

Your remark that she's treating the remains "like a souvenir from some trip" may be more apt than you realize. Actually, your parents did share a big "trip" together, and one of the partners is pining for the other. Your mother may find solace in having the ashes nearby. One woman I know replaced the sand in a large hourglass with her husband's ashes, probably for the same reason.

Share your feelings with your mother and ask about hers. Obviously, she's at ease with the ashes being close by. I doubt if she's interested in burial or scattering at this time. Maybe she'd like to keep the ashes until her own death, then have you mingle them with hers or place them beside hers in a colum-barium (a wall of small vaults into which urns are placed).

As a nursing professional, you're used to taking charge. But I'd like you to allow yourself the luxury of not "coordinating" this situation. This is simply about being a daughter whose fa-ther has died. He's close by but not in the form your aching heart wants. Allow the ashes of the body that used to hug and hold you to provide a little consolation now. ✏

Treating emotional symptoms

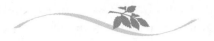

I'm caring for a home hospice patient who's terminally ill with gastric cancer. His physical symptoms are under control, but he seems to have a restlessness in his soul. When I ask if he has any unfinished business, he turns away without answering. His wife says she thinks he's thinking about a son from his first marriage. They had a falling out years ago and haven't spoken since. I don't want to butt in, but intuition tells me this rift needs to be resolved for his own peace of mind. What's your advice? — S.T., Ontario

I ADMIRE YOUR self-restraint. You might be tempted to telephone the son, but that would violate your patient's privacy and overstep your role, no matter how well intentioned you might be.

I suggest asking the patient's wife to join you at the bedside. Explain that you're aware of the break in his relationship with his son, then ask if he'd like to talk about it. Also offer to leave if he wishes to speak privately with his wife about it.

If he declines to discuss this with you, remind him that you care about his comfort, both physical and emotional, and that if he ever does feel like talking — about anything — you're available.

This isn't the time to gather up your sphygmomanometer and walk out the door. Instead, continue your assessment in a warm, dignified way while making small talk or discussing how much fluid he's been drinking. You want to promote a sense of acceptance and trust, regardless of whether he chooses to confide in you.

If, however, he rolls to face you and his wife and begins to share his feelings, sit down, touch his arm, and give him your undivided attention.

Recently, a lovely woman I knew only casually asked me to help with her terminally ill dad. Dana explained that the physician had said that her dad was depressed and had also recommended another round of chemotherapy. But her dad had turned down treatment for cancer or depression and seemed to be willing himself to die by refusing to eat or drink.

"Is anything else going on that could be making him feel so hopeless?" I asked.

Dana then revealed that her dad had left her family when she was a child. He'd come back into her life after her mom died 3 years ago. "It's kind of hard for me to let him go now that I care about him," she admitted.

"So you love your dad, Dana?" I asked.

"Yes, I guess I do."

"Does he know that?"

"I haven't said it in so many words, but I think he knows."

I suggested that she go in and tell him all the things in her heart. "Then we'll ask him what he wants," I said.

An hour later, I was paged to her father's room. "Oh, Joy" she sobbed. "I told him I loved him and forgave him. He opened his eyes and said, 'I accept your forgiveness, and I love you too.' Then he just rolled back on the pillow and died!"

I have to admit that I was a bit stunned.

"Dana, you gave your dad two wonderful gifts today: your loving forgiveness and permission to be relieved of his burden of guilt. This is powerful stuff."

She smiled and gave me a big hug.

I hope your work with your troubled patient is as rewarding for you. ❧

Walking on eggshells

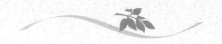

Should I encourage family members to say good-bye to a dying person who doesn't want to acknowledge his terminal condition?
—*J.B., California*

YES, BECAUSE otherwise everyone misses an opportunity for healing and growth that will soon be gone forever. My experience with Ed, a 47-year-old man dying of liver failure, is a good example of how a nurse can ease the way for a patient and family.

A fierce fighter, Ed couldn't admit that the battle for his life was almost over. He refused to talk with me about hospice or palliative care, saying only that he was going to beat this.

The medical and nursing team had informed the family that Ed was dying and they needed to gather round. They didn't think they could remain in the room without breaking down. His mother asked me to meet with the family, who felt as if they were "walking on eggshells" whenever they talked to him.

When the family had gathered, I said, "Dr. Mitchell has

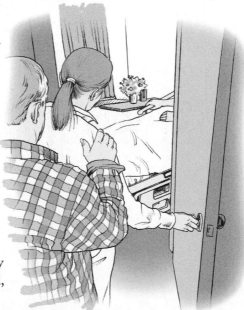

spoken to Ed about his condition, and I know Ed doesn't want to accept it. But we're running out of time and I believe that each one of you needs a chance to say good-bye and tell Ed how very much you love and value him."

Silence. I waited. Then Michelle, Ed's 17-year-old daughter, said softly, "I'm first." After she returned, her sister went in, followed by Ed's two brothers and his youngest daughter, Susan.

When Susan returned, she was crying. "He got real upset," she said. "He asked me why everyone was coming in like that. Then he said, "God, I must be dying! Am I dying?"

I asked her, "What did you say?"

"I told him yes! Then he grabbed me real tight and told me he loved me and wanted everybody to be with him."

The family rushed to Ed's side and gathered close, sharing their heartfelt thoughts with him. I can't help but think it made losing the battle a little less difficult for everyone. ✎

Everything's not okay

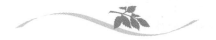

*I work in an oncology unit where many of our patients are
readmissions. One gentleman has been especially dear, and we're
all fond of him. He's been a trooper over the past 6 months,
tolerating nasty adverse reactions to drugs that aren't helping
anymore. I've observed him trying to share his feelings about
dying with his family, but they don't want to hear it. So he
accommodates them by pretending that "everything's okay."
How can we help this family?* — T.B., Michigan

FIRST, FIND 20 minutes to sit down quietly with your patient.
Arrange for colleagues to check on your other patients so you
won't be disturbed. Tell this gentleman about your observations and ask if he'd like to speak with you about his feelings.
He'll probably appreciate this opportunity.

Next, ask if he'd like your help in relaying some of these
concerns to his family. You might offer to speak with them on
his behalf, be present while he tells them his feelings, or
arrange a family-patient-physician meeting in his room. The
advantage to a meeting that includes the physician is that the
family can have all their questions answered at the same time.

Encourage your patient to ask his physician about discon-
tinuing treatments. For example, he might ask: "Doctor, do
you see my condition improving, staying the same, or worsen-
ing?" "Can you offer me any hope that the benefits of further
treatments will outweigh the side effects?" or "Do you think
it's reasonable for me to seek only comfort measures at this
point in my illness?" Gently ask him how he feels about the
frankness of these questions, how he thinks his family members will respond to the answers, and, most important, what he
wants now in terms of treatments and palliative care. If his

loved ones are too anxious to have this talk with the physician, you'll have an accurate picture of your patient's wishes to relay to them.

I recall working with a terminally ill woman married to a corporate president. We all thought he'd agree with her wishes to "just go home." Amazingly, he pleaded with the oncologist to do everything, even though the poor lady was fading into the sheets. I sat with him as he wept openly. He spoke of his mother's death when he was a little child. He was left alone in the house and told that "big boys don't cry" as his grieving father stormed out to the local tavern for a long night of drinking. Most of his young adult life was spent searching for the one woman who'd replace his lost mother. "Elaine is that woman, Joy," he told me. "I just can't bear to lose her too."

So it's important to let family members express what a loved one's death means to each of them.

You say the staff is fond of your patient. Imagine, if you can, the loss his wife and children, who've loved him for years, will suffer when he's gone.

The most important thing is to allow each person to speak his truth. But you must start with the truth about your patient's limited time left on Earth. ➤

Asking the impossible

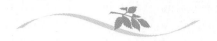

Just 2 years out of school, I'm working in a medical/surgical unit. I love my job. So what's the problem? My stepmother is dying of cancer and Dad and my two brothers expect me to give up my job to care for her. I'm feeling guilty because I don't want to do this. My stepmother and I are like oil and water, and I'm afraid our time together would be tense for both of us. What should I do?
—R.A., California

IF YOU'VE READ my past columns, you know I remind nurses never to "should" on anybody, including ourselves. So I don't even use the word in my vocabulary. However, I also want to remind you that no one can make us feel guilty; we give another person that power when we're afraid to say no.

Your stepmother is terminally ill, and you can't fix this. Explain to your father and brothers that you're perfectly willing to be available periodically to help out, but that they need to talk with her about having hospice as her main nurse provider.

You have every right to continue in your career and enjoy your calling. When you come home feeling rewarded for helping others, you'll be more willing to stop by and give a little to your stepmother too.

On the other hand, if you resigned your position, you'd undoubtedly feel resentful — and your stepmother would sense those feelings.

Let's also consider practical matters. Do your brothers and father think that you could do all the nursing care yourself? If so, they don't have a realistic idea of what's ahead. Explain to them that you'd need help from a hospice team — and from them too.

Sometime, when you have all the players in place and your stepmother is having a good day, you might sit down privately with her and talk about repairing your relationship. Let her take the lead and try to be open and compassionate. Who knows? She may use this time of her life to impart some wisdom that you can someday share with your many future patients. ❧

Devoted daughter

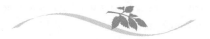

My sister, who's also a nurse, is taking care of our father. He's dying of stomach cancer and needs help with everything. She's exhausted, yet she won't accept my help. I really want to do things for her and for our father too. Do you have any suggestions?
— W.T., Arkansas

JUST ONE—let her do whatever she wants. I know it'll be tough. But for whatever reason, she's chosen this role for herself.

My guess is that your sister is trying to make up for some past negative feelings or actions by giving your father devoted care now. Because stomach cancer doesn't usually kill quickly, she may have the time she thinks she needs to repair any rifts.

Your concern could mean that you have feelings that need to be resolved too. But your sister isn't allowing you time or space to work them out.

Try sitting down and talking with her. You might be surprised by how many thoughts and feelings you have in common. Who knows? She might even confess that she really wants your help but she doesn't know how to tell you that she feels overwhelmed. Or perhaps she considers you to be your father's favorite; if so, she may be trying to win his approval—and yours.

Maybe, though, she feels what she's doing is nothing more than her duty as his daughter. That's okay too. She's a grown-up, and she's perfectly capable of making her own decisions. The worst thing you could do is to usurp her role "for her own good."

However, she shouldn't be caring for your father if she becomes too exhausted to give competent care. If that's the case, you'll have to step in. Tell her that she's doing a fantastic job and that you aren't taking it away from her. But let her know that you think what's best for your father is for her to get some rest and for you to pitch in.

Remember, *you* have a right to closure too. Take advantage of your sister's "break" to have some special time with your father.

Bury the hatchet

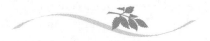

Although my parents separated 5 years ago, they never divorced. Now my mother is dying from emphysema and she wants Dad to be with her. I offered to move in with her instead, but it's my father she wants. Do you think this is a good idea? — *P.K., Missouri*

I'VE SEEN THIS type of situation before—sometimes it works, sometimes it doesn't, depending on how willing everyone is to let go of the past and focus on the present.

I once cared for a man with lung cancer who wanted to die at home. I shared this with his wife, who visited every day.

"Bill and I have had an extremely difficult marriage," she told me. "He drank a lot and abused me and the kids. I know this sounds awful, but I was relieved when he got too sick to hit us. I'll come here every day just as I've been doing, but I won't take him home. And that's that."

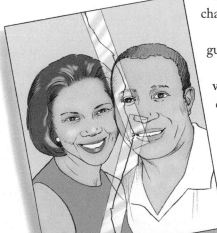

Her eyes dared me to challenge her. I didn't.

Bill died 3 days later. I guess he knew.

Another patient of mine was a retired air force officer. One year before he was diagnosed with liver cancer, his wife moved out of their home. She said she couldn't take his infidelity. Their three daughters took her side. But when Phil was hospitalized, they all visited and forgave him. He and Nettie even renewed their vows in his room.

Then we arranged home hospice care for Phil, and his "girls" took him home. A small pump continuously provided his swollen, jaundiced body with high doses of morphine to control his pain.

He'd been home 1 week when Nettie called to say he'd died.

"We all feel blessed, even in the middle of this tragedy," she said. "Before he died, Phil called each of us to his side and told us how sorry he was for all the heartache he'd caused. You know, we took him out every morning to sit in his Buick — even on the day he died. I'm glad we could do that for him."

I really can't say whether reuniting your parents would be a good idea — that depends on them. But I do know for sure that it's best to bury the hatchet before you bury someone you love.

Resist quick judgment

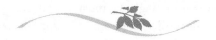

*My terminally ill grandfather has decided that he'll go to a
nursing home to die, even though I've told him that he can move
into my home. As a nurse, I certainly could give him the care he
needs. But more than that, I really want to spend this time with
him. What can I do to change his mind? — L.K., Wisconsin*

YOUR GRANDFATHER HAS been making his own decisions for
a long time. You'd be smart to let him continue doing so.

Your situation reminds me of Albert Barr, one of my patients.

"Early in June, my doctor did this surgery on my stomach,"
he told me recently. "But I couldn't eat, so about 3 months later he decided I'd have to go under the knife again."

I asked him how things turned out.

"Well, he couldn't do anything in there. He just sewed me
back up."

A few days after our conversation, the doctor decided that
Mr. Barr needed a feeding tube.

My patient was adamantly opposed.

"When a man can't eat his food the regular way, nature is
trying to tell him something," he said.

Because he was a retired infantryman, he asked to be admitted to the Old Soldiers' and Sailors' Home. We made the
arrangements. He was to be transferred a few days later.

His daughter, meanwhile, had asked him to come live with
her. He'd refused. I sat on the edge of his bed and asked him if
he'd reconsider her offer.

"No thanks," he said again. "I appreciate what she's trying
to do, but she has her own life to live. Besides, she's divorced

and trying to work and raise a baby on her own. No sir, I ain't gonna be a burden."

I told him that I thought he must have done a good job as a father to have instilled such strong values in his daughter.

"She loves you, Mr. Barr, and wants to spend these final weeks with you. Won't you consider the benefits of sharing this time together?"

"She can visit me at the home," he said.

"We can share then."

We both sat in silence. After a few minutes, he looked up at me. Tears streamed down his sweet face.

"My job was to sacrifice for my daughter so she'd have a better life than I did," he said. "Don't you understand? Going to the home is the only way I can keep giving to her."

I understood. This was an old soldier's final unselfish act. Later, at a moving family conference at his bedside, his daughter understood, too.

So, before you make a quick judgment, sit down and talk with your grandfather. Listen to his words, his reasons. Then make your generous offer one more time. If he still wants to die at the nursing home, remember that he has the right to choose.

And you can choose to accept his decision — unconditionally. ≋

Choosing the right time

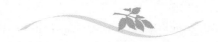

Although my terminally ill patient has some good days, I know he won't last much longer. Most of his family is here with him, but one son lives out in Wyoming. When is the right time for the family to call him? They don't want him to come here too soon. But they don't want to wait until it's too late either.
—*B.H., Pennsylvania*

I'M AFRAID there's rarely a time that's precisely right. But in my experience, most people would prefer to come early and have a few last days with their loved one, rather than arrive only in time for the funeral.

A few years ago, I had a dying patient who I thought had only a few hours to live. I called his daughters, who quickly arrived at the hospital. We kept a death watch for the rest of the day.

And the night…and the next day…and the next night.

Finally, on the third day, one of the daughters said, "I thought Dad was dying."

"He is," I replied.

"Well, when do you think he's really going to do it?" she asked.

He "really" did it later that afternoon.

For a minute, I chided myself for not being more precise with this family. Then I realized no harm was done. In fact, the daughters had 3 days to say their final, important words to their father. Yes, they'd lost some sleep and skipped a few meals. But, in return, they'd gained an experience that would comfort them for many years to come.

In your situation, what's the worst thing that can happen? The son comes to Pennsylvania to see his father, returns to

Wyoming, then a day later finds out his father has died? He'll probably be grateful for those last few days that he had with his father.

So, call your patient's son and give him all the information you have. Then let him make his own decision.

His agenda

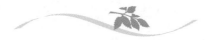

My 40-year-old son is dying of colon cancer. The irony is that I'm an oncology nurse, and I'd urged him to see a doctor several years ago when he began having problems. But he didn't think anything was wrong. So he procrastinated until it was too late. Now I'm so angry that I can hardly talk to him. How should I handle this?
—*L.T., Nebraska*

I'M TERRIBLY SORRY about your son's situation, but I'm sure you know that blaming him is both unkind and unnecessary. What do either of you gain?

Perhaps you're blaming yourself, thinking you should have made him go for help. Now you're not only grieving as a mother, but also you may be worried that, somehow, people will think you're not a competent nurse. But remember, your son is a grown man who makes his own choices and decisions.

Instead of focusing on your anger, I believe you need to think about your son now and find out—from him—what his agenda is. This is *his* experience, after all. I know you're suffering as you anticipate losing your son. But you aren't going to lose your life—your son is. What does he have to say about it?

Dying requires a lot of energy. I believe that every terminally ill patient should have a chance to talk about his feelings with someone who cares enough to sit and listen without interruptions or judgments. This doesn't require extensive interviewing skills—just genuine caring.

Can you do this for your son? Just tell him that you love him and care about what he's going through. Ask him what his life and death mean to him. I'll bet he has a lot of emotional string to unravel.

You could also ask him if he'd like to tell you why *he* thinks he's dying. Try not to make any judgments, though — don't let "would have" or "should have" creep into the conversation.

If you can help your son sort out and find meaning in his life, I'm sure that his dying will be easier. For both of you. ❧

Unraveling painful feelings

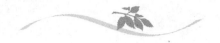

I've been a nurse for over 20 years, so I'm embarrassed to admit that I'm not handling my mom's terminal illness well. Almost every time I visit, she tries to give me a few pieces of jewelry or a scarf or a photo album. I keep refusing to accept these gifts because I don't want her to give up. Last week, she gave my two boys some mementos. When they showed them to me, I started to cry. I guess deep down I know she's going to die, but I'm just not ready to lose her. What can I do to handle my feelings better?—H.G., *Alberta*

FORGET ABOUT BEING a nurse right now and just be a daughter who's hurting. You've been a daughter longer than you've been a nurse. And your mother isn't your patient—she's your mom and your boys' grandma. No wonder you're so upset.

You might also be identifying with your own children and fearing that they must one day feel this pain when you're dying. So this is a complex experience. Just let yourself be in the moment.

Your question reminds me of a wonderful story titled "Annie and the Old One." An elderly Navajo woman works on a loom all day, weaving a woolen blanket. She tells her little granddaughter Annie that when she finishes it, her life also will be finished. At night, while the grandmother is sleeping, Annie goes to the loom and unravels the wool.

I think you're "pulling an Annie." And I don't blame you.

It's okay that *you're* not ready, but I think your mother is. Giving things away indicates closure. It also shows her affection for you and your sons.

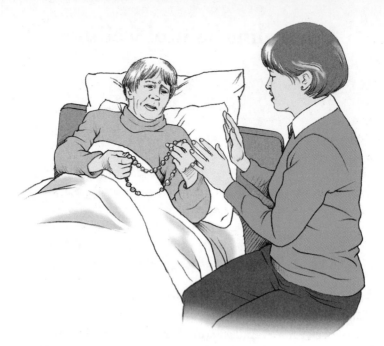

I'm glad she has the energy and love to carry out her own wishes, and I hope the recipients of her gifts will enjoy them and express their pleasure to her while she's still alive.

Remember: Feelings aren't right or wrong; they're just feelings. You were feeling sad and upset. You cried. That's honest.

Tell your mother and your little guys why you cried. That's being real. And you can't beat that. ❧

Choosing when to die

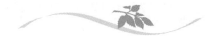

For 2 days, my father and I sat by my mother's hospital bed as she was dying. Toward the end of the second day, I persuaded him to go home with me to take a shower and change clothes. Unfortunately, Mom died while we were gone. Now Dad won't forgive me for encouraging him to leave her side. What can I do?
—D.K., Arkansas

I'M SORRY that your father is misdirecting his anger at you—after all, you're grieving too. His reaction is understandable, but I don't think it's justified.

Obviously, he agreed to leave. Although there's nothing wrong with wanting a break from a deathbed, he may be feeling guilty that he didn't sacrifice his own comfort to be with your mother. Maybe you feel guilty for taking a break too.

If witnessing your mother's last breath was important to your father, he needed to say so. We're all responsible for our own actions after all.

Could you possibly entertain the idea that your mother *chose* to die during your absence? Seneca, a Roman statesman and philosopher, said, "Just as I choose a ship to sail or a house to live in, so I choose a death for my passage from life." So we may actually participate in how, when, and where we leave the body.

You might propose this idea to your father—that your mother waited until he left to make her final exit.

Of course, he may be upset if he believes his lifelong partner "deliberately" died while he was gone. I've talked with survivors about this idea of a loved one making a choice to die. Some have accepted it, but others have been angry and have even questioned their worth as a mate—as if the value of the entire relationship hinged on the exact moment of death. So you might suggest that your mother chose to die when she did to spare the two of you pain. Remind him that the nurses were there, so she didn't really die alone.

I've had many experiences with patients who either held on or let go with undeniable participation — Leona, for example. This dark-eyed, raven-haired woman was dying of cervical cancer that had metastasized throughout her pelvis. She wanted to time her death for her son's arrival from Colorado.

"Bobby can't afford to drive all the way here just for a visit, Joy," she told me. "So I'm going to finish this while he's here so my funeral can get done with too."

And she did.

So I'm convinced that your mother left her body at the time she decided was best for her. After all, it was *her* death. 〜

4

Managing difficult situations

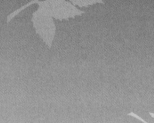

Hold that thought

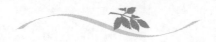

As a recent graduate, I thought that assessing patients would be easy because I'm a good observer. But when assessing my first patient in my new job, I was distracted by her roommate, who kept interrupting me with questions and irrelevant comments. She was receiving chemotherapy and looked very ill. How could I have handled this situation gracefully? —R.S., *Quebec*

LET ME ASK you, a good observer, this question: Which of the two patients needed you more?

Yes, the interrupting lady.

You say she looked sick and was receiving chemotherapy. I'll bet she was frightened and asserting herself to get your attention.

Recently, I was doing a pain assessment on a patient whose lung cancer had metastasized extensively. No sooner had I settled myself in a chair next to her bed when my patient swung out of bed, entangling me in a web of I.V. and oxygen tubing.

"I've got to go to the bathroom!" she exclaimed.

Quickly unplugging the pump and grabbing up yards of extended oxygen tubing, I followed her to the bathroom. She immediately expelled a loose bowel movement. I helped clean her and eased her back to bed.

I'd just settled back in the chair when my patient's roommate, Mrs. Howell, said, "This room stinks."

I excused myself from my patient, deodorized the bathroom, and closed the door. "There, I think that'll do the trick." I smiled at Mrs. Howell, then pulled my chair close to my patient's bed.

"Now," I said to my patient, "if you could please tell me on a scale of zero to…"

"That spray didn't do any good."

Mrs. Howell again. She continued to complain loudly, apparently determined to capture my attention.

Sensing that some deeper need was driving this behavior, I excused myself, went to the nurses' station, and quickly flipped to the progress notes and read "pancreatic carcinoma, extensive metastasis, prognosis grim. She is taking bad news well."

Maybe she's not taking it so well after all, I thought. She's terrified.

I returned to both of my patients. Taking Mrs. Howell's hand I softly said, "Mrs. Brisson is having pain, and I need to help her get relief. If you'll give me a few minutes I'll take good care of her. Then, if you'd like, we can talk."

Mrs. Howell nodded, squeezed my hand, and lay back on the pillows, visibly relaxing.

You may not find a terminal prognosis behind every example of demanding or manipulative behavior. But you will find a patient who's hurting and needs your nursing touch. ✎

Going the extra mile

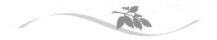

A patient died in our unit at about 6 a.m. His two sons, who'd stayed through the night, wanted to help carry his body out of the hospital to the hearse. But the nurse-manager who came on duty at shift change cited hospital policy and directed that the body be taken to the morgue. The night-shift nurses and I felt that this wasn't a very compassionate decision. What are your thoughts?
—*B.L., Florida*

ONE OF MY favorite sayings is "The best way to take care of your patient is to care for your patient." In the case of terminal illness, your "patient" is the patient *and* his family and friends. The "caring" doesn't stop when someone dies.

Your experience reminds me of a similar situation I was involved in years ago. I'd expected the patient to die during the night, so I said tender good-byes to the pastor-patient and his three sons. When I checked the room the next day, I found that my patient had died and that one son had chosen to stay with his father's body until the undertaker arrived.

We usually take bodies to the morgue so patients won't be disturbed by the sight of morticians coming and going. But this young man needed things done differently.

I sat with him and kept watch — an ancient ritual originally intended to prevent wild animals from devouring a corpse. He chatted lovingly about his dad, sharing stories of how he always wore a brown bowler hat and long overcoat in winter.

"Once, my dad drove for hours through a bad storm to visit a young prisoner," he said. "When he arrived, the guard told him visiting hours were over and he'd have to leave. Dad explained the long-distance drive and asked that he be allowed a brief visit and prayer. Again, the guard refused."

"You can see, Joy, that Dad is tall—6 feet 2 inches. So he slowly opened the car door and unfolded his long lanky self. Well, you can probably guess that Dad got his visit—and time for an extra-long prayer!"

We sat together, sometimes laughing, sometimes in silence, until the undertaker arrived. How sad it would have been to miss out on this memory-making exchange, a touching experience for both of us.

The next time you find yourself dealing with a death that requires you to go the extra mile, invite your manager to participate. She'll be richly blessed. ➢

Being there

I'm a clinical coordinator in a large CCU. Many staff members attend funerals of patients who die here. Because I'm in a leadership role, I feel obligated to go. But just thinking about it upsets me. At one funeral I attended, I became so distressed that I had to leave and sit in the car. I'm hoping you'll say that sending a sympathy card and a nice note is adequate. — *T.Y., California*

CERTAINLY CARDS and telephone calls are thoughtful, but I'd like you to consider the immeasurable gift of a "human moment." Giving your presence to the grief-stricken is more precious than you can possibly imagine. You're acknowledging that one of the members of our human family has been taken from us, and we're the lesser for his absence.

You don't have to spend a long time trying to impart wise words of comfort. A simple touch on the arm and a softly spoken, "I'm so sorry. Please know that you're in my thoughts" will suffice. People may not remember what you say, but they'll remember your presence. It says you were kind enough to stand in someone else's pain. That's what I mean by having a human moment.

Try not to be so hard on yourself. I'll bet your anxiety stems from the obvious reminder that you, too, must die. Or maybe you have a traumatic memory of a funeral you attended as a child.

I appreciate your concern and sense of responsibility. It's worth resolving these apprehensions before they prevent you from coping with a death closer to home. ✎

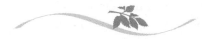

Man's best friend

I'm a nurse at a veterans hospital. One of my favorite patients,
who is quite open about being terminally ill, has told me that he
wants his elderly beagle to be put down and buried with him.
He says the dog, which he's had for 16 years, will be company for
him in the afterlife. Apparently he has no family or friends willing
to adopt the dog after his death.

As a dog lover, I'm uncomfortable with this. What do you
think? — *W.E., Pennsylvania*

YOUR PATIENT'S REQUEST harkens back to ancient ritual.
Speech is only about 3,000 years old, yet we know of graves
10,000 years old containing spears, primitive tools, seeds, and
animal bones.

This tells us that man has an innate need to find meaning in
death and to anticipate an afterlife in which the deceased will
live again with
needs and
wants similar
to those he
had while
alive.

Numerous
civilizations
have ob-
served this
custom of
burying objects
and animals with their own-

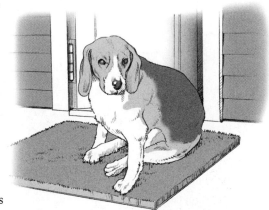

ers. Mummified cats have been found in the tombs of royal
Egyptians. Cats were revered in ancient Egypt, so we speculate

that they were killed at the time of the pharaoh's death to give him companionship in the afterlife.

Most veterinarians with whom I've spoken would hesitate to euthanize a healthy younger dog. However, if this beagle is over 16 years old and destined for an animal shelter after your patient's death, his wish might be honored.

You might feel better if you sit down with this dying man and ask him to share a story or two about his dog. This might help you understand what the dog means to him. To him, the thought of ending their time on earth together may be far more comforting than imagining his beloved pet spending its remaining days alone in a shelter.

Talking trash

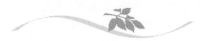

I work as a nursing assistant for a home hospice agency. One of my patients, Mrs. Howell, is an alcoholic dying from lung cancer. Every time I visit her, she's drunk and treats me rudely—swearing at me, refusing to cooperate, and ordering me around. Some days I just hate having to go there. How should I handle this? —M.B., Quebec

IT MIGHT HELP to remember that we die the way we live. Mrs. Howell has probably used alcohol to cope with life's challenges for a long time. Now that she's facing the biggest crisis of her life, she's resorting to her "old friend" to help lessen the pain.

You don't mention her family situation. I wouldn't be surprised if she's driven them away with her abusive behavior.

Sometimes when a patient acts obnoxiously, she's testing her worthiness to receive loving care. When you're the target, this behavior can cause you to feel angry, then guilty about your anger.

You don't have the option of abandoning her—you're ethically required to stand by your patient. (Remember the words of Dame Cicely Saunders, founder of the modern hospice movement: "If you don't have problems, you don't have a hospice.") But you're *not* obligated to take abusive behavior from anyone.

Seek assistance from your hospice colleagues. At a multidisciplinary meeting, talk about establishing some boundaries for your patient.

Establish a simple rule: There will be mutual respect during each visit.

Also talk about various tactics you could use to back up this rule. Some people favor a behavior modification approach: The minute she swears at you, you quietly leave. But I find this approach punitive. Plus, it may reinforce her low self-esteem, perpetuating her anger and aggression.

Instead of walking away silently, I recommend a direct and honest response: "Mrs. Howell, I'm here to help in any way you'd like, but I don't want you to swear at me." If you're kind but consistent about "calling" her on unacceptable behavior, you're likely to trigger some changes. If her behavior improves during one visit, bring her a special treat the next time. Before long, she'll grasp that you expect to be treated with respect.

Also discuss your patient's alcohol use with the hospice nursing staff. Could she be drinking more to relieve physical pain? Her nurse needs to assess whether she's adequately medicated and make changes in her regimen, if indicated.

You or the nurse may also want to discuss your patient's alcohol use with the patient and encourage her to limit her intake. Just be nonjudgmental and avoid lecturing. Expecting her to stop drinking isn't realistic, but your concern could encourage her to talk more openly with you about her feelings.

Whatever your approach, don't expect huge changes. But I'm betting that deep down, Mrs. Howell wants you to like her and appreciates your help. She may never say so, but I suspect she looks forward to your visits. Sounds to me like this lady could use visits from the hospice coordinator, clergy, and a social worker too.

A lock of silver hair

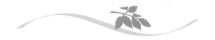

*In our ICU, we've had to handle several sticky situations
involving visitors. More than once, for example, a fiancé has
arrived as an ex-spouse was leaving. How should we screen these
visitors, especially during the patient's final hours?*
—*H.G., California*

I BELIEVE THAT anyone the patient wants present should be
invited. If the patient can't voice his request because he's unconscious or deeply sedated, the people who love him must be
offered a chance for a last visit or to say good-bye.

During a patient's final hours, I consider the ICU to be neutral territory. Each visitor has a unique relationship with the
dying patient, and incomplete closure can profoundly affect the
family and patient.

When family and friends gather, I look for the person
standing to the side of the group. Many times, this person is a
disenfranchised griever who needs special attention, someone
who's stepped aside to allow the dying man's children or siblings to take their "rightful" places at the deathbed.

I observed this scene a few weeks ago. The woman in this
case was my patient's "friend" of 2 years. After becoming a wid-
ower, Mr. Kraft needed someone to look after him and prepare
meals. Love blossomed and the two became a couple and lived
together, but never married. After suffering a cerebral hemorrhage at home, Mr. Kraft was rushed to the hospital, intubated,
and admitted to the ICU. His prognosis was poor.

Two days later, his children decided to remove him from the
ventilator. He was given morphine and extubated. Surrounded
by loved ones whispering their farewells, Mr. Kraft was unaware of his companion's tears. She was leaning against the

sink, arms folded across her chest in a self-hug. I asked if she'd like to speak to Mr. Kraft. She nodded a grateful yes.

I escorted her to the head of the bed. Several others stood back to make room. I told her, "I like to think that he can hear, even though he can't respond. Just tell him whatever you want. Do you need privacy?"

She slowly shook her head no and gave a little smile. She never spoke. She just smoothed his silver hair. Over and over. Tears flowed onto her cheeks, but she never wiped them away.

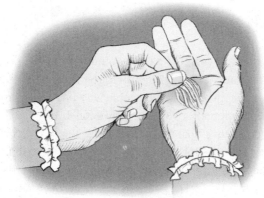

After a few moments, Mr. Kraft's breathing stopped. And so did the smoothing.

Later, the family gathered at the elevator. I asked if anyone would like a lock of Mr. Kraft's hair. His lovely lady was the only one who said, "Yes, please." ✎

Dealing with a stillbirth

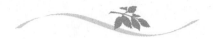

I work in a labor and delivery unit. After a stillbirth or the death of a newborn, we offer the parents photographs of the baby, his baby cap and blanket, and his ID band. We also refer them to the appropriate support group. Do you have any other suggestions for supporting parents in this sad situation? —M.B., Pennsylvania

NOT LONG AGO, I attended a neonatal bereavement seminar at which Dr. Ida Martinson, one of my nurse-heroes, spoke. Among the many points covered, she discussed two areas of rights that you and your colleagues might want to consider. First are the rights of the dead newborn. According to Dr. Martinson, the baby has these rights:

+ to be recognized as a person who was born and died
+ to be named
+ to be seen, touched, and held by his family
+ to be buried with dignity.

In Dr. Martinson's view, the baby's parents have these rights:

+ to see, hold, and touch their baby
+ to have a photograph and (possibly) a plaster cast of the baby's hand
+ to receive mementos such as the crib card, ultrasound picture, and a lock of hair
+ to name the child and have cultural and religious practices respected
+ to be cared for by an empathetic staff who will honor the parents' individual requests
+ to have time alone together
+ to plan the farewell rituals and burial.

This is such a sad time for everyone—parents and staff alike. I hope these suggestions help.

Don't use the empathetic lie

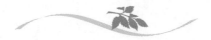

Working on an obstetric unit is an upbeat experience—unless I have to care for a mother whose baby has died. Then, I'm so uncomfortable that I hurry through her care so I can get out of her room. I know she needs more support from me, but I don't know how to give it. —J.L., New York

WHENEVER I'M CALLED to the obstetric floor, I know it can mean only one of two things: a dead baby or a dead mother. I dread that call, because I'm not too brave about either.

I remember Elizabeth, who'd had five stillbirths. Her sixth pregnancy seemed to be going well, but in the seventh month she had another stillbirth. When I visited her after the delivery, we wept together. Then I asked her if she wanted to see her baby. She did, so I offered to go downstairs to the morgue and bring the baby back up to her. But she wanted to go to the baby. "I'm ready. Just get the wheelchair," she said.

I wheeled Elizabeth into the pathologist's air-conditioned, carpeted office—a softer environment than the morgue—and left to get the baby. "Would you like to be alone with her?" I asked when I returned.

"No, would you please stay?" she asked.

I handed her the baby. Elizabeth pulled back the blanket to see her daughter, then started rocking and crooning. "What's her name?" I asked.

"Jessica," she whispered, but she wasn't talking to me.

Later, after I'd taken Elizabeth back to her room, I felt sadness mixed with pride. I'd helped her, through sensitivity and genuine concern. I assumed nothing. I gave her control over her situation...tragic as it was. I asked her what *she* wanted to do, then complied with her request. I let her be my teacher.

Elizabeth taught me a valuable lesson: You can never say to a patient, "I know what you're going through." Some people call this statement the empathetic lie because you can't possibly know what another person is feeling.

So, acknowledge that. And be ready to listen to a mother put into words the hurt she's feeling. ✎

Topsy-turvy world

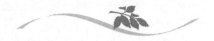

*My sister-in-law has breast cancer and is receiving chemotherapy.
She's lost most of her hair, she's had bouts of nausea and vomiting,
and she feels tired most of the time. I'm very concerned about her
7-year-old daughter, my niece Angie, who's been acting nervous
and frightened. My brother says she cries when he's firm with her
(especially about eating breakfast and taking her vitamins) and
that he has to force her onto the school bus in the morning. The
whole situation is breaking my heart, but what can I do?*
— W.A., Pennsylvania

YOUR BROTHER IS probably overwhelmed, and your sister-in-law is just trying to get from one day to the next. No wonder your niece is frightened — she's trying to figure out who's in control and who'll keep her safe. An immediate family talk is in order.

You don't say whether Angie knows about her mother's diagnosis. If not, she must be told by people who love her. If she does know, she needs to talk — she's obviously very scared.

I notice an interesting correlation between your sister-in-law's symptoms and Angie's morning behavior. Your sister-in-law can't eat because she's nauseated; your niece's refusal to eat her breakfast mirrors her mother's distress.

You or your brother might call the oncologist and ask for an antiemetic and for tips to improve your sister-in-law's appetite. If you can make her more comfortable, Angie will feel better too.

Also consider why Angie resists taking her vitamins. Is she afraid of them? Although she probably didn't think twice about swallowing them in the past, everything in her world is topsy-turvy. She can't trust any medication now—what if it makes *her* hair fall out?

So give her the facts. Tell her that the medication her mother takes is strong so it will kill the cancer. But Angie doesn't have cancer, and her vitamins won't make her feel bad.

Give her some positives too. For example, reassure her that her mother's hair will grow back and that her mother will be able to do "mommy things" again when she feels better. (Of course, I'm assuming that your sister-in-law's prognosis justifies this statement—you wouldn't want to hold out false hope.)

Then encourage your brother and sister-in-law to snuggle up with Angie and ask her what frightens her about school. I'll bet that she isn't afraid of school itself. She's probably fearful that things at home might get worse while she's away. If Mommy dies, Daddy might fall apart. Who would be there to make sure she's okay?

This is a perfect time for you to show your support and caring. Tell Angie that you're quite healthy and strong and that you can help her and Daddy until Mommy gets better.

Just remember that Angie is like anyone else in a family affected by cancer—she's afraid that she won't be taken care of and that her life isn't going to be the way it was before her mother got sick.

All of you need to be open and honest about your feelings. Hug each other and draw on the hidden strength in your spirits. The bottom line is that Angie needs to trust the adults in her life and to feel sure that they love her.

Even if Angie's cry for help is what prompts your family talk, I'm sure everyone will benefit. ✎

Loaded questions

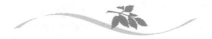

One of my patients has already had a long, painful battle with cancer. Now he's unresponsive and on a ventilator. His wife is trying to decide whether to continue aggressive medical treatment. Last night, she pulled me aside and asked, "What would you do if he were your husband?" I felt put on the spot and didn't know what to say.

How should I handle questions like this in the future?
—J.W., British Columbia

I RECENTLY participated in a family conference in which a physician was asked the same question. I think she handled it well. Let me share the story with you.

Mr. Johnson, who'd suffered a devastating stroke, was unresponsive and ventilator-dependent. His wife and two adult sons gathered in a conference room to discuss his condition with his oncologist, neurologist, and me. As we took our seats, I chose to sit among the family so all the "white coats" didn't appear adversarial or threatening.

Dr. Anderson, the oncologist, began with a brief review of Mr. Johnson's history and current status. She was kind but firm in her opinion that he'd never return to his original self.

Matt, the younger son, confronted her with a challenge: "Isn't it wrong in medicine to say 'never'?"

Dr. Anderson blushed slightly but remained respectful and professional. "You're right. Perhaps that wasn't the best choice of words. I meant to say that the chances of your father having a full recovery are miniscule."

"We're not talking about him having a full recovery. We want him any way we can have him!"

Dr. Bushnell, the neurologist, spoke of his third neurological assessment and said that 90% of patients in Mr. Johnson's condition do survive.

"See, Tim, Dad could pull through," Matt said to his brother. "But you want to pull the plug."

"Only because that's what he told me he'd want." Tim turned to his mother. "He said he told you too, Mom. Do you think I *want* him to die?"

Dr. Bushnell quickly clarified his point. "About 90% of these patients survive, yes. But most live in nursing homes, unaware of where they are and needing round-the-clock nursing care. I doubt your father will ever even recognize you again."

I entered the fray by saying, "We're always interested in anything the patient might have said about what his wishes would be in case something like this should occur."

"Dad didn't want to be kept on a machine," Tim said again. His mother tearfully nodded.

I continued, "I think we'd all agree that there are worse things than death, and this man was saying that he'd prefer death to living the remainder of his life unconscious and hooked up to a ventilator."

Dr. Anderson had started to add her support to that thinking when Mrs. Johnson interrupted. "Let me ask you this, doctor."

I knew what she was about to say.

"What would you do if this were your husband?"

Talk about a loaded question. Although we want to answer our patients' questions honestly, a frank reply to this one would taint family decision making by putting the weight of a professional's personal opinion on one side or the other. I held my breath.

Dr. Anderson stared straight ahead for a moment. The room was silent.

Then she spoke. "I can't answer that. Only you can make this decision based on what your husband's wishes are in the context of the information we give you."

I slowly let out my breath as Mrs. Johnson slumped back in her seat. "I guess that's it then," she said. "We ought to do what he'd want." Both sons nodded. From then on, discussion centered on the process of removing the ventilator and keeping Mr. Johnson comfortable through the dying process.

When I left that night, I thought that Dr. Anderson had hit exactly the right note when she responded to Mrs. Johnson's question. She'd gently reminded them that every situation is unique and that only those involved can make the "right" decision. ❧

Human moments

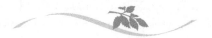

Last week a physician wrote an order directing "social services to discuss hospice with patient." Nothing in the progress notes indicated that the physician had discussed the patient's prognosis with her. I felt uncomfortable with this request, so I phoned the physician. He didn't take my call, but his receptionist said, "The doctor wants you to arrange for inpatient hospice because the family can't take care of the patient anymore."

I don't feel qualified to have this kind of discussion with a patient I barely know. Should this be my responsibility?
—C.P., Virginia

DISCUSSING HOSPICE CARE entails discussing the prognosis. That's the physician's job, not yours. The patient may have questions about treatment options that you can't answer. Check your job description and the policies and procedures for case managers. Ask your nurse-manager to intervene if necessary.

Arranging for palliative and hospice care requires a dialogue that no one really wants to have, physicians included. But our patients and their families deserve nothing less.

I was in a similar situation when a young physician, Dr. Hall, wrote an order for me to talk with his patient, Jane Lee. He not only wanted me to discuss hospice placement, but he also wanted me to inform her that it wasn't cancer that was killing her, but heart failure.

Believing he was better qualified than I to discuss her medical condition, I declined to act as his surrogate but offered instead to accompany him to her bedside. I pulled a chair up to the bed for him. He reached out and gently held Jane's hand. But when he told her that she couldn't go home, she abruptly withdrew it. She was obviously overwhelmed.

"I thought you said the cancer wasn't so bad right now," she said.

"Yes, well, no," Dr. Hall stammered. "What I meant was, it's your bad heart that's the problem now. Your breathing has gotten much worse even with the medication and increased oxygen."

She lay back and shut her eyes.

Dr. Hall started to get up, but I gently pressed my hand on his shoulder, pushing him firmly into the chair. I spoke softly. "Jane, Dr. Hall cares about you, and all of us feel terrible that we can't fix this. You may ask either of us any questions about anything."

I felt Dr. Hall tremble slightly, but I wanted him to realize that words are the most powerful tools a physician has. When such information is given poorly, his patients will never forgive him. But when bad news is given well, his patients will never forget him.

Finally, Jane opened her eyes and took Dr. Hall's hand. "I don't blame you, you know. I just hoped I'd have a little more time."

"I'm so sorry," he said.

I left the room. Dr. Hall, the physician, had invited Kevin Hall, the human, to his patient's bedside. What a fine team they made.

Masking the pain

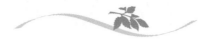

My husband is a doctor. Several months ago, a friend of ours who was also a doctor died in a boating accident. His widow stays in her robe all day and rarely leaves the house. Several times she's called my husband and asked for sleeping pills. The first time, he prescribed a few Restoril tablets but he doesn't want to give her any more. What can we do to help our friend? —R.G., Florida

I RECENTLY READ about a similar situation. Two doctors died in a small-plane crash, which also killed the pilot and copilot. Because the doctors' widows were financially secure, they had the "luxury" of remaining recluses. The other two widows had to find work to support their families. In contrast to the doctors' widows, they lived a more structured life with responsibilities that demanded focus for a certain segment of the day.

You don't need any more details to grasp my point: Sometimes life forces us to pull from our marrow the grit to get up and get moving. Obviously, your friend can't do this right now.

What she needs to do is tell the story of her tragedy over and over again as a way to process her grief. Can you sit with her, allow her to sob and scream at God? Can you just hold her?

Your husband is smart not to overmedicate her. One of the tasks of mourning is to feel the pain of the loss. Too often, grieving people believe they can recover from a terrible time if they mask the pain with medication for several months. They think that when they stop the drugs, healing will have magically occurred. Instead, the pain comes back more fiercely than ever.

Remind your friend that there's no right way to grieve — there's only her way. And that's the best way for her. ✒

The key: Understanding

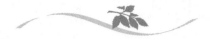

My aunt lives on the other side of the country and has no family close enough to provide daily care. She's terminally ill with cancer and has inquired about hospice. The director of the program told her she would have to have a relative or friend actually live in the same house with her to qualify under the admission policy. Is this true? —A.E., RN

UNFORTUNATELY, SOME hospice home care programs require a caregiver to live with the patient, even though my experience has shown this is unnecessary.

But I do believe in having a "designated" caregiver — an individual who doesn't have to live in, but agrees to be responsible for checking on the daily progress of the patient. In some situations, this caregiver could simply be a neighbor, a private duty nurse, or the entire bowling team.

A few years ago, I worked with an elegant lady who had lived alone all of her adult life and demanded to die that way. Inez had enough money to hire nurses around-the-clock but chose not to do so. She wanted to be alone, except for the periodic visits by the hospice team.

We complied with her wishes, even to the point of hanging the key to her front door on a long string. The visiting nurse would ring the doorbell, signaling Inez to lower the key out the window beside her bed. After admitting herself into the apartment, the nurse would replace the key in preparation for the next hospice visitor.

It was my honor to sit beside Inez as she quietly laid down her *Time* magazine and died. But even if she had died alone, I don't consider that to be the worst thing that could have hap-

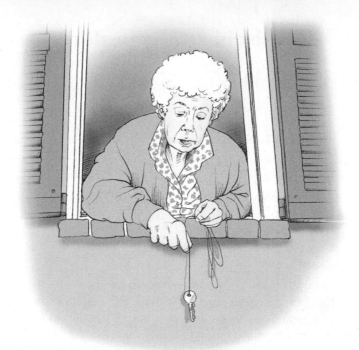

pened. The worst thing would have been for our organization
to require her to change her lifestyle to receive services.

Too many vulnerable folks have been visited by "goody two-
shoes" community service agents who make value judgments
about how and where patients should live. They're quick to
yank people out of their homes and place them in extended-
care facilities or in-hospital units. They're seeking to fill only
their own needs. But dying people have the right to die their
way. Whatever way that might be.

One of my hospice patients lived alone. She drank large
quantities of whiskey. She died alone, having fallen down the
cellar steps. The manner of her death saddened me briefly, but
then I found quiet pride in knowing I'd defended her right to
live and die her way.

I'm positive now that it matters more how we die than that
we die. 🙖

Knowing when to stop

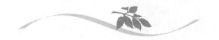

My 7-year-old Joshua was diagnosed with leukemia when he was 4. He seems to have had every treatment possible, and now I think maybe we should stop. I just don't want to give up too soon. How can I make the right decision? —K.S., Pennsylvania

I CAN'T IMAGINE how difficult the past 3 years must have been for you. Knowing when to stop aggressive therapy is a tough call.

Although many professionals disagree, I feel the first step is for the doctor to speak honestly with the child and tell him that the treatments are no longer working. Then he and the parents should allow the child to choose whether or not to continue.

I was privileged to care for Danny, a child the same age as your Joshua. He also had leukemia, and I knew he wouldn't survive.

I spent as much time with Danny as I could—I'd fallen in love with the little guy. I brought kittens from my home to his hospital bed, and I took him outside in his wheelchair to throw stones in the river or wade in the fountain near the courthouse. I grew quite fond of his family too—especially his mother Nancy, who was always honest with him.

One afternoon Danny asked his mother, "What are they gonna do next? Are they gonna give me more treatments?"

"There aren't any more treatments, Danny," she said.

He paused, then said, "I want to go home."

So we piled all the gifts and cards and equipment into the car and took him home, to his own bed. I went too, keeping watch with his parents for 2 days and 2 nights. We gave him the only thing left to give—tender, loving care.

Moments before he died, his mother told him to put out his left hand and let Jesus hold it. "I'll hold your right hand so you'll always have someone holding you."

I've witnessed hundreds of deaths, but Danny's was the best — Nancy was honest and honored his wishes.

So my advice is to talk with Joshua's doctor. Ask him to give you all the facts about your son's prognosis. Then ask him to discuss the situation with Joshua so he can find out what your son wants. When he knows, all three of you should sit down and decide how to proceed.

No matter what Joshua wants, remind him that you love him and you'll certainly miss him. Then tell him that you'll hold his hand if he wants to let go. ✎

Quitting too soon?

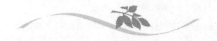

My 7-year-old nephew, Mark, is terminally ill with rhabdomyo-
sarcoma. His mother abandoned the family when he was a baby,
and my brother has raised him alone.

When I visit Mark in the hospital, he waits until we're alone
to ask me questions about other boys and girls who are "like me."
Last week, he told me he thought the physicians were running out
of ways to help him. I've explored with my brother the idea that
it might be time to stop these terrible treatments and take Mark
home. He said he wants to, but he's afraid he'll feel guilty for quit-
ting too soon. As a nurse and a concerned family member, how can
I help these two fellows, whom I dearly love?
— G.C., North Carolina

PLEASE KNOW of my heartfelt concern for you right now. Suffering certainly has taken several forms in this sad situation.

The dilemma your brother faces is one experienced all too
often by parents of terminally ill children. I think the answer
lies in including the child in the decision making.

This requires utter honesty, and not many families, physicians, or nurses are eager to walk that walk and talk that talk.
Yet as far back as the 1970s, pioneers like Elisabeth Kübler-
Ross and Myra Bluebond-Langer showed us that children can
be quite knowledgeable about their impending death.

But we still need to be aware of the child's fears. Like anybody else, children are fearful when they feel helpless or powerless. This might tie in with Mark's questions about other children "like me." He may be wondering what happened to them.
(Did they die?) He might also be trying to validate his own
suffering by exploring whether the others found meaning in
their ordeals.

Because children fear abandonment or separation from loved ones, explain to your brother the terrific support home health care hospice can provide as well as your commitment to help (if you so choose). And let Mark know that you and his daddy will be with him throughout the remaining days of his life.

Finally, children fear punishment—especially when it seems unfair. This may be the concern Mark expressed when he tested you by saying that he thinks the physicians are running out of ways to help. Maybe he's really asking, "Why more painful, useless treatments?"

Mark trusts you and probably sees you as his advocate. He knows you'll take his words to his father. It seems to me that the little patient knows it's time to stop.

If he says he wants to go home, assure him that in place of treatments, he'll receive medicine to keep him comfortable. Remind him that if he wants to return to the hospital, he may.

As Mark finds relief in this honesty, he'll begin to offer more of his thoughts and feelings. All the adults in his world must be willing to accept whatever he needs to express. When you and your brother can do this, Mark will be able to find meaning in whatever time he has left to live. Seeing the potential for peace in this child's passing can ease a bit of the fear your brother has about quitting too soon. ✎

Should they shield their son?

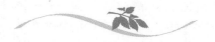

Last week, our daughter died of a respiratory infection 3 days after her birth. Our 2-year-old son knew that he was going to have a little sister. Now, we don't know how to tell him she died. What should we do? — *K.T., Washington*

THE WHOLE FAMILY, even a child, is affected by a tragedy like yours. One woman told me after her baby's death, a teacher tried to console her 7-year-old son. When the teacher said she was sorry that his mother's baby had died, he responded, "It's *our* baby that died."

I don't think you should try to shield your son from the news. I'm sure he senses your grief. Not knowing what's wrong is scarier for him than learning the truth. I suggest that you and your husband sit down with him and tell him gently and honestly that his sister won't be living with you. Don't hold back the tears.

Because of his age, he may not comprehend the finality of death. He might ask you when the baby will be coming back or when you'll get another one. These questions can be quite painful. Again, cry as much as you need to, and hold him tight. Give brief, simple, honest answers to his questions. If he has trouble understanding the concept of death, you might compare this one with that of a flower or little animal.

Try not to say "we lost the baby." He may worry that you'll "lose" him, too. And he might wonder why you aren't trying to find the baby. But don't worry too much about finding the right words. The most valuable thing you can give your son is love and honesty.

Children are resilient. I bet your boy's need for comfort will help you and your husband through this painful time. ✑

The right to grieve

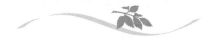

Yesterday, my uncle died of a myocardial infarction. He was my mother's only brother. She's in a nursing home, and my father doesn't want me to tell her what happened because he's afraid the news would upset her too much. She's always been sickly and rather fragile emotionally, so I can see his point. What do you think we should do? — D.L., Colorado

YOUR MOTHER HAS a right to know about her brother's death. Not because he was her only brother, but because he was such a part of her life.

I'm appalled that anyone would think he has the right to withhold information that affects another person's life. And I'm tired of hearing the lame excuse, "We thought you needed protecting." I hope no one ever second-guesses for me.

Assuming that you know how another person will react is nothing short of manipulation. What about your mother's right to grieve? She needs to share this time of mourning with others. She might want to attend her brother's funeral — even if she's ill and frail. Would you deny her that opportunity?

The bottom line is that your mother can't make the best decision for herself unless she's given all the information. Tell her gently, then be prepared to answer her questions and to discuss her feelings. Share your own sadness, and encourage your mother to reminisce about happy times with her brother. Ask her about some of her favorite childhood memories.

I don't want to sound disrespectful, but your father has to realize that human beings are tough creatures. Certainly, hearing about her brother's death will upset your mother. You can expect her to cry and to be distressed.

Don't be afraid that the bad news will kill her. She may become depressed, lose interest in eating, and choose to stop living — but the emphasis is on "choose." I believe that we fully participate in when, how, and where we'll die.

Hurry to your mother. Take her hand and tell her you have some bad news that will hurt her.

Then stay with her and ask, "What would you like to do, Mom?" ✎

No experience necessary

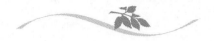

I'm concerned about one of the families I care for in home hospice. Only 47, the patient just learned he has extensive cancer and has chosen not to receive chemotherapy. Although shaken by the bad news, his wife and sons want to care for him at home until he dies, and he says that's what he wants too.

The problem? I'm not sure the family is up to the job. His wife, who has health problems of her own, seems frail. His two sons, who are only 18 and 21, have never experienced a death in the family.

Should I suggest inpatient hospice so they'd all be more comfortable? I just want to do what's best for everyone. — G.F., Ontario

YEARS AGO, we didn't have hospice nurses…just each other. I believe that taking care of each other is part of our nature. So isn't your role to support families as they do the only thing they can do for each other?

It may be humbling for us professionals to face, but the best "nurse" for an individual is someone who loves and adores him. We can always teach a frail wife how to turn her bedridden husband; she already knows compassion and advocacy.

Pushing the right buttons

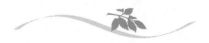

I'm a medical/surgical nurse. Amazingly, the nurse-manager in my unit looks and acts like my sister, who died 2 years ago of alcoholism. This may sound cold, but I never liked my sister. And now I can't stand to be around this manager. She pushes the same buttons that my sister did. I'm considering transferring to another unit. Do you think that will get rid of this ghost? —A.L., Nevada

FIRST, THE BAD NEWS. We create the "buttons" that other people push. No one can *make* us feel good or bad. We give others that power when we seek approval and validation from them instead of listening to ourselves.

I'm sorry you had such a difficult relationship with your sister. Her death must have been especially hard on you. As a nurse, you knew the poor prognosis for your sister's alcoholism and self-destructive behavior. But the sibling in you felt the loss from deep in your marrow.

I'm wondering if you're feeling guilty for not "changing" your sister and saving her life. You might also feel somewhat relieved that she's out of your life forever.

I don't know why you and your sister weren't close. But you can heal that relationship now, even though she's dead. Forgiveness can be a one-person act. All you have to do is to let go of the anger and the "shoulds." Simple, but not easy.

A friend of mine, Bob, was extremely disappointed that his father wasn't more loving and caring. When Bob's father was dying of cirrhosis, I encouraged Bob to write to his dad expressing *all* of his feelings. (Feelings are neither good nor bad; they're just feelings.)

So Bob wrote a letter, but he felt let down because he never got a reply. His father died several months later. "See," he said

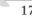

harshly to me. "What good did it do? My old man acted just like he has all of my life!" I reminded Bob that his goal in sending the letter was to express his feelings. True forgiveness requires nothing of others.

The best way to forgive the dead is to just do it. It can work with your manager too. Certainly, you can transfer to another unit or another hospital or even another state. But ghosts, as you said, tend to follow and haunt us.

So I advise letting go from your end; the folks on the other end don't have to do or say anything.

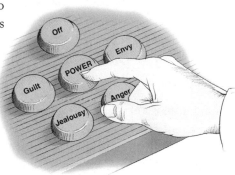

Push your power button. Send your sister and your manager peace and light. See them happy and smiling. Genuinely wish them love and joy. See them receive it from you with open hands.

Then look out, my friend, because your spirit is going to feel the magic. And I bet you're going to want to push that button again. ✑

All in the family

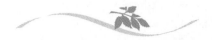

I'm a nurse-manager struggling with a large family keeping vigil over a dying patient. Although they're quiet and respectful they're spilling out of the patient's room, clustering in the hallway, sleeping in the family room — in short, taking up every square inch of the place! When I asked them to visit a few at a time in shifts, they seemed offended. How can I regain control of my unit without appearing insensitive? —F.R., *Missouri*

I BELIEVE YOUR need to "regain control" of your unit may be at the root of your struggle. Your patient's family is also seeking some control in frightening circumstances. They can't control when their loved one will die, but they can choose to be where she is. It doesn't matter whether she's in the hospital or at home in her own bed. When they can be at her side, they're not only "there" for the dying woman, but they're also "there" for each other.

I'm sympathetic about the intrusion upon the normal flow of your unit. But this isn't a normal time for this family. They're losing someone they love forever. The deathwatch eventually will come to an end. In the meantime, you have an opportunity to be a hero to the family and a leader for your staff. Ask your patient relations or guest services department to provide extra coffee, soft drinks, and snacks. Get extra linens and pillows. Guide other visitors to waiting areas unoccupied by crying family members. Open an unused conference room for them and provide pagers similar to those used by some ICU or OR families.

Be creative and empathetic. Your patient's family will never forget your kindness. ✎

Abandoning the vigil

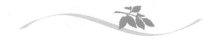

I'm a private-duty nurse who cares for many terminally ill patients. Usually I encourage family members to remain at the deathbed. But recently, one patient's daughter became so distressed that she rushed out of the house, upsetting the rest of the family. Should some people be discouraged from attempting to maintain a deathbed vigil? — P.D., Ontario

I'M CAUTIOUS ABOUT "shoulding" on people, especially during such emotional times. Each person brings her own baggage to this experience, with personal expectations about how the event will evolve. She also has an idea about what her role will be: caregiver, silent observer, or take-charge leader. When asked to be or do something outside of that self-assigned role, she's likely to become anxious.

Support and encouragement from someone like you can ease that anxiety and create a safe space. But some people, for whatever reason, simply can't keep the vigil. Their stance may be difficult for other family members and even the dying person to understand.

But this isn't about understanding; it's about accepting. The person who just "can't" be there needs permission to be somewhere else. Then the deathbed can be a place of just loving, without anyone feeling she needs to change who she is or what she's feeling. ✎

Someone's waiting for her

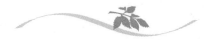

I'm a family practice physician and my wife's a surgical nurse.
I've read your column and wonder what you think about a
patient's participation in his own death. I don't mean someone
who commits suicide, but one who wills himself to die.
—*D.B., British Columbia*

ACTUALLY, DOCTOR, I believe that all patients live or die in
spite of our care. (That's rather humbling to those of us in
nursing and medicine.)

Many times I've seen patients choose to finish their lives
rather than go to a nursing home, endure another amputation,
or continue with futile chemotherapy. We all need a reason or
purpose to wake up every morning. No one can give that to
another.

Last week, one of my favorite physicians shared a story with
me. As an intensivist, Dr. Peters was caring for a 91-year-old
woman who'd had an episode of heart failure. As she typically
does with ICU patients, Dr. Peters spoke to Mrs. Dobbs about
her wishes regarding heroic measures.

"Oh, don't worry about that, dear," said Mrs. Dobbs. "I
signed my living will and all of that business is taken care of."

Dr. Peters assured her patient that her wishes would be honored. Then she added, "I want to tell you that you're doing better, so we really don't need to dwell on that."

"Oh, but you see, dear, I have someone waiting for me,"
replied Mrs. Dobbs. "Mr. Dobbs has been gone for years. I
miss him and I want to see him."

Dr. Peters nodded respectfully but again reassured Mrs.
Dobbs that her condition was improving.

Later that evening, Mrs. Dobbs began singing "Amazing Grace." She asked her nurse to join in, which she did. As another physician entered her ICU cubicle to assess her, Mrs. Dobbs waved him away. "Don't come in now," she said. "I'm focusing."

A few hours later she complained of "pain all over" and the nurse administered morphine. A short time later, Mrs. Dobbs left this world. She'd already explained why: She had someone waiting for her. ✎

Accent the positive

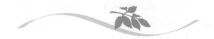

Last week, a patient who was dying of lung cancer told me she regretted not doing anything meaningful with her life. I didn't know what to say. Do you have any thoughts on how I could respond if anyone else asks me that question? —*J.T., Arizona*

WHEN A TERMINALLY ill patient says something like that to me, I try to help him sort out what was outstanding in his life.

Margaret, who had 19 children, was one such patient. She was dying of bowel cancer that had slowly spread through her pelvic area.

After I administered a morphine injection, she sighed and said she felt her life was ending prematurely. I gently took her hand and asked her what she meant by that.

"I have a big regret," she said. She eased herself over on her side and looked straight into my eyes. "I always wanted to be a nurse. But instead of going to nursing school, I got married when I was 18 years old, then started having babies. Now, here I am, dying, and I never got to be a nurse."

We sat quietly. I waited patiently for her next words.

"It isn't that my life is wasted," she said slowly. "It's just that being a nurse was something I wanted to do when I was younger and now I'll never get the chance to do it."

I had an inspiration. "Wait a minute, Margaret. Doesn't a mother wash and diaper and feed babies?"

"Of course," she answered.

"And, as a mother, don't you clean and bandage cuts and scrapes?"

She nodded.

"And, as a mother, don't you help kids with broken arms and bloody noses and loose teeth…?"

"And teach them about nutrition and health," she chimed in.

"Right!" I exclaimed. "See, those are many of the things nurses do. You just limited your practice to your home instead of a hospital."

As the morphine took hold, she lay back slowly on the pillows and closed her eyes. She held my hand tightly, gratefully. Then she fell asleep.

She died that evening surrounded by her husband and 19 children, all praying together.

Like Margaret, many of my patients have found solace in reviewing the highlights of their lives, with the accent on their contributions to others. Helping your patient see her life positively may be difficult, especially if she's depressed. But through gentleness and sensitivity, it can be done.

Keeping a secret

My aunt made me promise not to tell my uncle that she's dying of liver cancer. (He does know that she's not well, of course.) I'm afraid he's going to be shocked when she dies. What do you think?
— *C.N., Montana*

I THINK HE probably already knows.

Your question reminds me of a lovely lady I knew who was dying of lung cancer. She kept smiling despite the pain, although sometimes, between smiles, she'd cry about having to die, having to leave life.

I saw her husband once, when he brought her to my office for an appointment. He sat quietly in the waiting room, hat in hand, head bowed. She'd told me that she didn't think he knew how sick she really was.

He knew. He never said much, but I could see it in his eyes.

When he called to tell me that she'd died, I asked about funeral arrangements. "I'm finding little notes all over the house with directions and instructions on what to do and where to go," he said. "I guess she's still taking care of me."

Somehow, I think she always will.

Perhaps your aunt feels she's taking care of your uncle with her "conspiracy of silence." I believe that this is very important to her.

But your uncle *does* know how sick she is. He's protecting her by allowing the pretense to continue.

It's best not to interfere. ✍

.5.

Advocating for patients and families

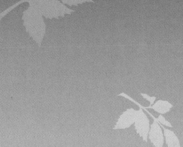

Fighting over futile care

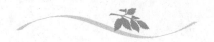

I'm an RN and my husband is a community representative on the ethics committee of a local hospital. Recently, we discussed the case of an unresponsive woman dying of cardiac problems. Her daughter wanted everything done, in spite of the physician's advice that the patient's condition wasn't treatable. The daughter refused to agree to do-not-resuscitate (DNR) status for her mother, but the physician wrote a DNR order anyway. Now the daughter is threatening to sue the physician and the hospital. How likely is she to win? — *L.L., Nevada*

I KNOW OF no case in which a hospital and physicians were found liable for stopping treatment over the objections of family members.

Please hear me clearly when I say that I'm terribly sorry when a loved one will die if cardiac or pulmonary arrest is untreated. But many of our patients die despite heroic treatment. Patients who have grave conditions are going to die, regardless of interventions. It's such a waste of valuable time — for closure and meaningful goodbyes — when family members spend a patient's final hours fighting in vain.

I'm currently involved in a similar case. The wife of an incompetent, terminally ill patient has repeatedly refused to agree to a DNR order. The physicians and consultants have all tried to get her to agree to no extraordinary measures. They each documented their conversations, then one of them wrote a DNR order. The legal justification is "futility of care."

The *Journal of the American Medical Association (JAMA)* offers guidance regarding hospital policies that allow DNR orders despite family refusals. One recommendation is to allow physicians to write DNR orders over family objections if the following criteria are met:

✦ The patient lacks decision-making capacity.

✦ The burdens of treatment clearly outweigh the benefits.

✦ The surrogate doesn't give an appropriate reason for heroic measures.

✦ The physician has made serious efforts to communicate with the family and to mediate the disagreement. (*JAMA*, 264[10]: 1281-1283, September 12, 1990.)

Certainly I feel compassion for any person losing a loved one. But acting isn't always appropriate just because modern medicine gives us the ability to act.

My approach in cases like these is to continue speaking with the distraught family member and ask what it means to have his or her loved one die. Inevitably, the reluctant family member says something like, "I'm waiting for a miracle" or "I'm not ready to let him go." These reasons are moving, but they don't warrant a resuscitation attempt when that action can't reverse the underlying medical condition.

In the final analysis, we have to be advocates for the patient who can't speak for himself.

Worth the risks

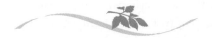

A dying patient was recently put through painful tests that I felt were unnecessary. As a recent graduate, I wondered whether to speak up or not. Now I feel guilty that I didn't. I guess I'm not as assertive as I could be. How can I improve? — B.N., *Pennsylvania*

I UNDERSTAND your situation. But, as you know, one of your roles as a professional nurse is to be your patients' advocate. That requires two things: knowledge (a professional responsibility) and assertiveness (a moral responsibility). By studying, passing the state board examination, and gaining experience, you become more knowledgeable. Your knowledge isn't worth much though, if you can't use it to ease your patients' pain and to improve the quality of their care.

You need to be confident enough to put your knowledge on the line — to say, "I know what's best here, and I'm going to express that opinion."

Recently, I cared for an elderly woman dying of lymphoma. She agreed to a course of chemotherapy to appease her daughter, who was also a nurse. After a week, my patient's white blood count was dangerously low and she'd developed sepsis.

One morning during rounds, I found her comatose, with a low blood pressure and faint pulse. Her breathing was shallow but not labored.

I asked her daughter and son, a pastor, about their wishes for resuscitation. They talked quietly with each other, asked my opinion, then decided to let her die a natural, dignified death.

I told the attending doctor of their decision and asked her to write a do-not-resuscitate (DNR) order. By this time, the patient was in a deep coma and barely breathing.

Immediately, the doctor told the son that she was going to order X-rays and blood work, then begin I.V. antibiotics. I couldn't believe what I was hearing. The patient was about a half hour from death, her children had been fairly well reconciled to that, and now the doctor was about to drag in the big guns.

I took her out into the hallway and explained the family's wishes. She agreed to write the DNR order, but said she was obligated to find and treat the infection.

"I agree," I said, "when there's hope of saving the patient. But Mrs. Bishop is going to die this morning."

"How do you know?" she snapped.

I put my knowledge — 15 years working with death and dying — on the line and said, "I know because of my many experiences watching the dying process."

She said nothing. But she didn't order the X-rays, blood work, or antibiotics.

We gathered the family together. I was deeply moved as Mrs. Bishop's son read the Psalms through his tears and her daughter folded her mother's hands across her chest.

My assertiveness was worth it. Really, I don't have any more of it than you. You just have to be willing to take risks.

Go for it.

One last shot

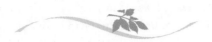

In our oncology unit, many patients are admitted for end-of-life care. Our staff collaborates with staff from our excellent hospice program, which is affiliated with the visiting nurse association. The problem? One oncologist admits terminally ill patients who seem unaware that they're dying. Instead, they think they're in the hospital to "give it one more shot." These patients are overloaded with I.V. fluids and even tube feedings and wind up suffering needlessly. How can we help them? — G.G., Oklahoma

I SEE NOTHING wrong with admitting dying patients to the hospital for pain management. But this oncologist sees death as a failure rather than a natural part of life. So he and the patient never discuss considering alternative plans, "in case this cancer gets ahead of us." The patient and his family are swept along in this physician's denial and unreasonable expectations.

Palliative care specialists know that overloading failing systems with I.V. fluids and tube feedings causes third-spacing and edema. By impairing breathing, pulmonary edema only adds to the patient's suffering.

Just as you have guidelines for giving chemotherapy, you need guidelines for admission criteria and care of terminally ill patients. If the oncologist isn't following facility policy, you and your nurse-manager should ask the chief of medicine to step in. If your facility doesn't have a current policy for terminally ill patients, work through channels to develop one. Encourage participation from everyone involved in the care of these patients, from social workers to ethics committee members. Be especially attentive to the advice of those who "do it right" — hospice and visiting nurses and physicians who specialize in palliative care.

Speak up!

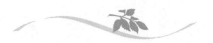

One of my terminally ill patients suffers constantly because her doctor won't prescribe morphine. He says that if he prescribes a narcotic, she'll know her bowel cancer has spread and she's dying.

I'm shocked that he would allow a patient to suffer needlessly simply to conceal her prognosis from her. I'd like to speak up, but I'm afraid I might get into trouble. Any advice? —*L.D., Delaware*

WHEN IN DOUBT, risk it! This patient needs an advocate. So, my advice is to speak up, loud and clear. If the doctor won't listen, talk to your manager. Insist that she relay your concerns to the chief of staff if necessary.

Next, talk with your patient. She knows she isn't getting better, whether the doctor has told her or not. Explain that her pain *can* be controlled and that she can change doctors if she's unhappy with the level of pain relief she's getting. Then, give her the names of three competent, compassionate doctors who could help her.

If you don't speak up, you may regret it later. Once, when lecturing at Tulane School of Medicine, I came across a nurse who was haunted by something she hadn't done for a patient. She urgently requested to speak.

She fervently told her story of being a young graduate nurse working on an obstetric floor. A woman, close to her own age, had delivered a baby girl, her second child. Unfortunately, the mother was hemorrhaging to death.

She pleaded with the nurse to bring her 2-year-old son to her so she could see him one more time. The nurse told the dying patient she would like to help, but she couldn't. "Children aren't permitted on the obstetric floor," she told the mother.

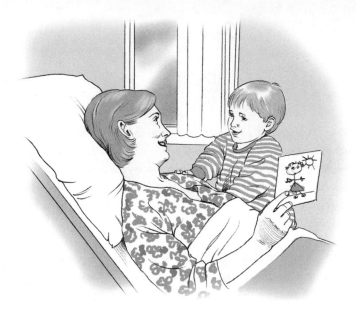

The event, you see, had taken place 45 years earlier. The nurse was still so haunted that she needed to "confess" to several hundred people.

So, don't delay any longer. Allowing this woman to suffer until she dies is the worst thing you could do. And you don't want to be regretting it 45 years from now.

Morphine on target

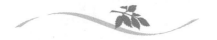

Recently, I cared for a patient with prostate cancer who had severe bone pain. His physician had ordered oxycodone and acetaminophen (Percocet), but it wasn't effective. When I asked the physician to order morphine, he refused. I'm wondering if my suggestion was sound—and if so, how to work with this kind of physician.
— C.C., New Mexico

BECAUSE PAIN FROM bony metastasis is usually severe, your request for an opioid was on target. You'd also want to add a nonsteroidal anti-inflammatory drug such as naproxen (500 mg P.O. twice a day) to reduce "hot" inflammation. This addition might also reduce your patient's opioid requirement.

All this advice is worthless, though, if the physician won't order the medications. To convince a reluctant physician, I determine how much analgesia the patient received in the past 24 hours and review nurses' notes to determine the number of times the patient requested pain medication and how he responded. Most important, I do a pain assessment with the pain expert himself: my patient. Armed with this information, I inform the physician of the patient's painful situation and request either an increase in the dosage or a different regimen.

If he resists, I press on with clinical specifics about the patient's condition. For example, I'll say "He's in such pain that he won't go to physical therapy for his hip exercises." The clincher might be something like this: "We won't have to call you tonight if we can get him comfortable this afternoon."

If all else fails, I go up the chain of command to the chief of medicine. And remember, all patients have the option of changing physicians. 〜

"Pink wheelchair" syndrome

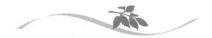

As a home hospice care nurse, I see how dying patients benefit from receiving care at home during their final weeks of life. Shouldn't we encourage all families of terminally ill patients to consider this option? —L.F., Tennessee

LET ME ASSURE YOU that I'm a great advocate for home hospice care. But before you promote it too emphatically, consider these important principles:

✦ Hospice isn't for everyone.

✦ The unit of care is the patient *and* family.

I've known many patients who were being cared for quite beautifully by family and friends and needed little help from professional caregivers. Yet I've also encountered situations in which home health care just wasn't viable.

I was taught by British physicians about the "pink wheelchair" syndrome, which involves family members who resist all efforts to move the patient back home. No matter how many potential problems professional caregivers offer to solve, the family always has one more objection. Finally they say, "But you don't have a pink wheelchair!"

My experience with Mr. Dalton is a perfect example of why some families need an alternative to home hospice.

Mr. Dalton, a 92-year-old Englishman, had moved to America 5 years earlier to help his daughter establish a small farm. His physician wanted me to ask him about his wishes to have palliative radiation for an ethmoid tumor.

I found Mr. Dalton sitting in a lounge chair. His long, white hair was combed straight back. I introduced myself, then asked if he felt like talking about his condition.

He replied with a Cockney accent, "I don't think I'm gonna survive this, am I, miss?"

"No, sir; it's an especially nasty brute."

He began speaking of his wife, Evie who died the day after Christmas last year.

"I miss her very much, miss," he said, now crying. "It won't be the worst thing if I just pass over soon."

As I do with all my dying patients, I asked what he wanted now that he was seriously ill.

"I'd like to go back to my daughter's farm and spend my last days with my grandson."

Our conversation turned into questions of logistics. His daughter worked, but her live-in boyfriend didn't. Mr. Dalton assured me that his grandson and family, who lived near his daughter, could visit daily.

I telephoned his daughter, relayed our conversation, and asked about her feelings regarding her father's wishes.

"Well, it's impossible to take him home!" she exclaimed. "I have a full-time job and farm work in the evening."

"I understand from your father that your son and his family live only 20 minutes away and might be willing to help," I replied.

"They're never around!"

"Well, we could have the hospice team in daily for several hours and the volunteer could — "

"He needs more than several hours," she interrupted. "Besides, I couldn't sleep at night, worrying that he's downstairs bleeding to death. I couldn't live with that."

I finally began to hear her.

"I suppose he also told you about my boyfriend," she continued. "Bert wants no part of this."

I got the message and realized I was dealing with the pink wheelchair syndrome. None of my solutions or expertise could allay her real concerns.

"Colleen," I spoke softly and clearly. "I hear your concerns. It's okay. We can look for placement in an inpatient hospice or in a nursing home that contracts for hospice visiting nurses. How do you feel about that?"

Silence. Then crying.

"I feel so guilty about not doing what Daddy wants, but I'm just so exhausted. When I come in tonight I'll talk with him."

Mr. Dalton was disappointed, and so was I. But experience has taught me not to force family members to do something they're not prepared to do.

Patient knows best

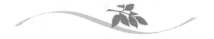

I'm a hospice home health care nurse working with a patient who's dying of cancer. He admits he needs our services but refuses to let us get him a hospital bed. During my last visit, he was having trouble breathing. I administered oxygen, as ordered, and added more pillows to help him sit erect. Before leaving, I offered once again to order him a hospital bed, but he adamantly refused. Driving away, I worried that I should have been more insistent. After all, it's for his comfort—and isn't that what hospice is all about? —G.A., Tennessee

YES, HOSPICE IS about comfort. But more important, it's about control: the patient's desire to control some aspect of an uncontrollable situation.

It's also about choice. Individuals afflicted with a disease that will ultimately take their lives are given the choice of hospice services. (They should be given all the information they need to make the best choice for themselves.)

I don't know why your patient refused the hospital bed, but I'll bet he associates it with his death. If he admits that he's ill enough to be in it, then he must really be terminally ill.

You offered. He refused.

He knows why. Do you?

Some hospice nurses might argue that you needed to discuss briefly the physiology of his breathlessness, then describe how the bed could be raised to make him more comfortable. They might even go so far as to suggest that you order the bed, based on your experience as a hospice nurse.

"You'll see, Mr. Markum, you'll feel better." But *who* will feel better? You?

You did well to administer the oxygen. I'd also suggest working with the hospice physician to plan a medication regimen that will make him more comfortable. For example, oral morphine every 4 hours could ease his dyspnea. You might also want to have some lorazepam (Ativan) on hand in case he becomes more anxious or restless—but no hospital bed unless he asks for it.

You're in his home—that makes you his guest. True, you're also a visiting nurse with good experience and training. Let's add sensitivity and understanding to the mix…and maybe another pillow. ⬿

The canine caper

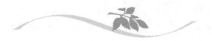

A terminally ill patient on my unit asked to see her dog one last time. When my manager said no, the patient was crushed. Do you think we should do this favor for her? —*L.K., Ontario*

YES, I DO, because she's making a legitimate request. First, find out why seeing her dog is so important. Take that information to your manager and explain the situation. Then, you and she should get together with other people at the hospital, including the infection-control nurse, and see how you can grant your patient's request. My point here is if you believe in helping her, put your beliefs into action.

I faced a similar situation at the hospital where I work. Although I don't recommend what I did as a routine course of action, here's what happened:

A dying patient wanted a last visit with her dog, Ruff. She'd had him for 11 years, since he was a puppy, and this was their first separation.

I talked with her son, who told me Ruff had been howling for his "Gran." Bringing the dog in for a visit seemed like a splendid idea to him.

At the agreed-upon time, we covered the 40-pound dog with a light cotton sheet and carried him into the hospital through the ED. He seemed cognizant of his mission and behaved in a gentlemanly manner. We managed to reach the patient's room undetected.

When we placed Ruff on his mistress's bed, we had to restrain him from climbing up to lick her face. But soon he was content to rest his head on her leg as she stroked him.

She spoke to him in their secret language, and she told him that they'd be separated again. But that didn't taint the joy of their brief reunion.

When it was time to go, my patient felt along the dog's noble head and face one last time. "Good-bye, Ruff," his mistress said.

I escorted her son and dog out, then returned to my patient's room. Her condition was deteriorating rapidly, and she died later that week.

I drove out to the son's house with his mother's few belongings. He gave her bathrobe to Ruff and told him that Gran had died. Ruff took the news well. He grabbed the robe and rolled around with it, then fell asleep within its folds.

You see, that last visit is important — for your patient and for her friend. I don't doubt that you'll benefit, too. ✎

Rushing rounds

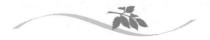

I work in a busy medical/surgical unit where certain physicians visit patients briefly, then quickly leave the room before we can even clarify scribbled orders. Recently, the family of a dying patient complained that the physician never even entered the room — but just stood in the doorway! After answering a few questions, he turned and scurried away. Is there anything we can do to fix this problem? — R.T., Georgia

THESE DAYS, most hospitals adhere to the patient's bill of rights, which guarantees, among other things, the patient's right to have information about his condition. If a physician won't take the time to meet this basic right, the patient is entitled to find another physician who will.

As your patient's advocate, speak up. Tell the physician about the concerns the patient and his family have expressed. If he still won't make time to talk with them, get your hospital's patient advocate involved and remind the patient and his family that they have the right to change physicians. You might also suggest that they inform their insurance company of their dissatisfaction: Some physicians become more responsive when their pocketbooks feel the pressure.

I witnessed a similar example of "rushing rounds" when keeping watch over a frail old gentleman in end-stage heart failure. Entering the room, I realized immediately that Mr. Philmore was close to death. I gently informed the family and gathered chairs for them around the bed.

No sooner were they settled for the deathwatch when the referring physician bustled into the room, booming a greeting and plowing across the family's feet and legs to get to the bedside. In a flash, he pulled the dying man forward, placed a

---

stethoscope on his back, then commanded: "A nice, deep breath now, please."

After a moment, he announced, "Well, you sound better. You're going to be all right." Then he bounded away.

I hurried after him. Without slowing down, he gave me an impersonal smile and said, "Give him whatever you think. I'll sign for it." Dumbfounded, I returned to Mr. Philmore and his family.

Mrs. Philmore asked if what the physician had said was true and I shook my head. Then I said, "If it's important to you to be with your husband during his last hours, I suggest that you stay close." Mr. Philmore died several hours later, with his family at his side.

Nurses often have to pick up the pieces of these unfortunate scenarios. We work with what tools we've always had: honesty, integrity, and compassion.

We have to have the courage not to abandon our patients to caregivers who seem to consider death a failure. I wouldn't trade these "failures" for anything in the world. ✍

Dumping ground

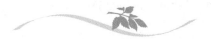

My sister has lung cancer that's metastasized to her brain. She started having seizures and dragging her right leg a couple of weeks ago. Months have passed since her last course of radiation therapy, and now the doctor says there's nothing more he can do. She's just going to get worse and die soon anyway, he says. As a nurse, I'm aware of my sister's poor prognosis. I can't help feeling that the doctor is dumping her. What can I do? —H.P., Colorado

I'M NOT SURPRISED by what's happening to your sister — I've heard many doctors say they couldn't do anything more for a dying patient. I imagine your sister's doctor is having trouble shifting to palliative care. Up until now, he's focused all of his energy on curing her.

Palliative care requires expertise, just as any specialty does. Crucial to this care is letting the patient know that the health care team is committed to supporting him for the rest of his life.

Right now, I'm working with a patient, Phil, whose doctor understands this. Phil's condition is similar to your sister's. His lung cancer was initially treated with surgery and radiation. About 10 months later, he began to have neurological symptoms and lost the use of his right hand and foot. The doctor ordered a brain scan. As he suspected, the lung cancer had metastasized to Phil's brain.

A month or so later, after more radiation, Phil began having seizures. The doctor prescribed Phenobarbital and instructed him to keep in touch daily. So even though Phil was frightened, he felt connected to his doctor. That alone relieved much of his anxiety.

A few more months went by. One day, I heard someone limping toward my office, then a feeble knock. When I opened the door, Phil stumbled into my arms. "Help me," he stammered.

Another brain scan revealed swelling around the tumor. The doctor ordered steroids, which seemed to magically reduce the swelling and symptoms.

But a brain tumor is real, not an illusion, and some of Phil's symptoms are slowly returning. The doctor and I met with Phil and his wife. We were honest with them, telling them that we couldn't cure the brain tumor but that we could continue to treat the symptoms so he'd be as comfortable as possible for the rest of his life.

That's the key phrase — *for the rest of his life,* no matter how long or short it might be.

So although we know that this brain tumor will eventually cause Phil's death, we're going to help him find comfort and dignity until that moment arrives.

Phil isn't dead yet, and neither is your sister. She deserves to be under her doctor's *care.*

You and she need to talk with him. Let him know that her needs aren't being met, and remind him of his obligation to her. Then ask him if he's willing to provide the kind, palliative care I've described. If not, tell him that you'll look for a doctor whose practice routinely includes palliative care. (But don't burn any bridges — your sister might need him to treat any symptoms that develop before she finds a new doctor.)

If he can't recommend someone else, you'll have to do some legwork. Check with your local hospice or a social worker at the hospital, read the hospital's doctor-referral directory, or talk with other nurses you know. Just keep looking. I know many doctors would be honored to get involved in your sister's care. ✑

Taking time for the "quiet visitors"

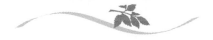

I work in an oncology unit where weary family members and close friends often maintain a vigil for dying patients. Sometimes they seem so lost and bewildered. What can I do to help them?
—*T.G., Oregon*

I APPLAUD your sensitivity. In a busy unit, that middle-aged daughter sitting quietly in the corner can be easily overlooked. Yet a simple gesture like resting your hand on her shoulder or offering a cup of tea might mean more to her than you could imagine. You might also call your hospital's guest services or patient-relations office and explain the situation. This intervention could trigger a visit from a member of that department who'll be able to support family and friends throughout the hospitalization.

You can also help by arranging accommodations for family members who want to stay overnight in the patient's room. A rollaway bed is the best option, but you can offer a recliner in a pinch. Be sure to provide extra blankets; air-conditioned hospital rooms can get frigid.

Encourage stressed and anxious visitors to ask any staff member for whatever they might need. Requests could be as simple as help in preparing special foods for the patient or as complex as placing calls to the Red Cross to arrange a compassionate leave for a relative in the military.

I'm well aware that most of your shift is spent providing acute nursing care. Thank you for your compassion for the quiet visitors who can be easily overlooked in the midst of a busy day. ✍

Against the rules

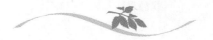

I'm an RN with a home heath care hospice agency. Recently I cared for a woman who'd had a long battle with metastatic lung cancer. After she died in her home, I asked her husband if he'd like to help carry her body out of the house to the hearse. The funeral director protested, claiming that this was "illegal." Later, he complained to my nurse-manager, who told me not to mention this option to families. I feel that this gesture is helpful to some grieving families. Do you agree? — H.G., New York

I CERTAINLY DO. The funeral director was off base — it's not "illegal" to have loved ones help remove a body form the house or hospital. Maybe he's concerned about possible liability issues if a member of the patient's family gets hurt while helping. (You could check with your state's Funeral Directors Association to find out what they advise.) However, I suspect the real reason for his objection was that he's uncomfortable participating in an act that's outside the norm to him.

Perhaps adhering to "the rules" helps him cope with the death and bereavement he sees every day. But any rules about grieving should be established by the mourners, according to what's most comforting to them.

Bearing the body is a step toward closure. Many times I've not only offered this activity to family, friends, and lovers, but also encouraged it. Not everyone wants to participate in transporting a loved one's body from the house, but that should be their choice to make — not yours, mine, or the funeral director's.

I can still remember the sister of one of my patients at our hospice house, struggling with the dead weight of her beloved brother as she helped carry him from his room to the waiting hearse. She held her head high, proud to participate in this last act of hands-on caregiving.

We don't dictate our patients' wishes — we ask them what *they* want to do. And we must do the same for our patients' survivors — they too are our patients.

Ask your manager to reconsider her decision. ☞

Worlds apart

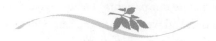

I'm caring for a Korean woman who's docile and soft-spoken. She denies pain from her bone metastasis, but I can see pain in her eyes. I don't want to harass her by continually asking if she's in pain, but I know she must be. Please help me help her.
— *M.P., California*

YOUR PATIENT'S response to pain most likely reflects her cultural values, which may be difficult for a nurse rooted in our culture to grasp.

At a time when American women are becoming more assertive, many women from other countries are still second-class citizens. Even those who live and work in the United States may continue to follow long-held cultural mores, which may include a reluctance to speak for themselves.

Recently, I was asked to visit Corrine, a woman from the Philippines, who was dying of breast cancer that had metastasized to her lymph system, lungs, brain, and pancreas. Her husband was sitting by the bed, speaking softly about the flight to Manila he was planning. A young white woman sat in a chair in the corner. She looked angry.

I introduced myself and told them that my primary concern was for Corrine's comfort. The young woman immediately leaped from her chair and shook my hand.

"My name's Ruth," she said. "I'm glad you're here to help." I later learned that Ruth was Corrine's sister-in-law.

I turned my attention back to Corrine, who looked tense with guarded positioning.

"Corrine, how's the pain?" I asked.

She turned silently toward her husband. He said her throat was burned from radiation treatments and it was too painful for her to talk or swallow. (I made a mental note to call her physician for lidocaine HCl [Xylocaine Viscous].) She was receiving 2 mg of morphine through a fragile peripheral vein in her left hand.

Once again, I addressed Corrine. "Can you just nod your head? Are you having pain?"

Ever so slowly, she nodded yes.

"Okay," I said. "I'm going to telephone your physician and ask that we increase the morphine so you'll be more comfortable."

Her husband, Joseph, shook his head. "We don't want any more because it will make her too sleepy," he said. "In 3 days, we're going to the Philippines."

I was amazed. "Oh, do you have a medevac airplane reserved?" I asked.

"No," he said. "I just told them we'd need a wheelchair."

At this point, Ruth spoke up, saying that Corrine was worried about the pending trip.

I asked Corrine if she wanted to fly to the Philippines. She stared right through me. No reply.

Ruth then suggested that we chat briefly in the solarium. When I excused myself, Corrine gave me a piercing look. Unfortunately, I couldn't read her wishes.

Talking with Ruth, I learned that a few weeks earlier, Corrine had told Ruth that she was tired of being sick and in pain and was ready to let go. She didn't want to make the long trip back to the Philippines.

"It's a 24-hour flight, Joy," Ruth explained. "I'm exhausted when I fly back to visit my in-laws— and I'm healthy! How is she ever going to make it?"

I explained that my first priority was to get the patient much more comfortable. "Let's just take this one day at a time," I said, knowing that Corrine probably had only a few more days to live.

Outside Corrine's room, I explained to Joseph that if we managed his wife's pain more effectively, she'd get more rest.

"I'll need three or four days to assess how the small increase is working," I explained.

"Okay," he said. "So we can plan on going to Manila by next week?"

"We'll see how your wife is doing by then," I replied gently.

We three gathered around Corrine's bed as Joseph spoke with her in Tagalog. I couldn't understand his words, but I did understand the success of my advocacy when Corrine looked at me with her beautiful dark eyes. She held my gaze, smiled slightly, then closed her eyes in relief.

Corrine and Joseph never made that flight together. But I did help get Corrine out of the hospital and back into her own bed, where she received home hospice care. She died 9 days later. Fortunately, because Ruth had told me of their private conversation, I could support her true wishes.

A similar strategy might help your Korean patient. Try to find an "Americanized" Korean friend or family member who could encourage her to be honest about her pain. Ask the attending physician to add a nonsteroidal anti-inflammatory drug to improve pain control without increasing sedation. (nabumetone [Relafen], 1,500 mg, is excellent.)

Offer the medication to your patient and explain why the drug was ordered and how you think it will help her. Then allow her to choose.

Whatever she says, accept her decision. If she refuses the medication, offer alternatives such as ice, acupressure, or relaxation. And add a large dose of loving acceptance. ✍

·6·

Mastering patient management

Minding your (bedside) manners

Recently, my mother died in the small hospital where I work. During the last few days of her life, when I remained by her side almost constantly, I noticed the nurses providing my mom's care didn't always have very good bedside manners. Sometimes they talked over her and didn't do any of the little extras, like fluff her pillows or brush her hair. Could you please address this in your column? — S.P., Nova Scotia

MANY YEARS AGO, when I was in nursing school, we performed nursing procedures on one another before inflicting our neophyte skills on our patients. We were injected (I.M. and S.C.), bathed, turned, and kept N.P.O. I believe those experiences made me sensitive to what patients go through and helped me become a gentle and compassionate nurse. This sensitivity can be learned, and we must teach one another.

I encourage nurses to do the following when caring for a dying patient:

✦ Use a soft voice, both with the patient and the family.

✦ Move slowly and gently about the room. Avoid bumping the bed, dropping side rails, or slamming doors.

✦ Don't yell back at the intercom. Whenever possible, quietly excuse yourself and go to the desk to respond.

✦ Tidy up the patient's immediate area, removing all unnecessary linens and supplies and wiping up the overbed table. (Gosh, this sounds like a job description for a 19th century nurse!)

✦ "Inform" before you "perform." For example: "Mrs. Ross, I'm going to gently wash your face now."

✦ Use warm water for bathing and a bath blanket to protect the patient's privacy.

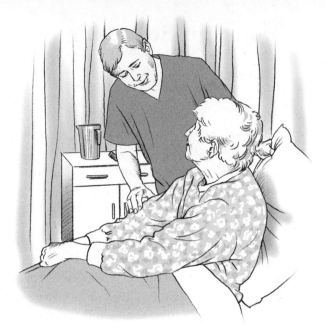

✦ Change linens frequently and use lots of pillows for special positioning.

✦ Don't leave the television blaring all day (unless, of course, your patient wants it on).

I'm especially particular about mouth care. Loving friends and family may be reluctant to get close to whisper good-bye if the patient's mouth and breath are unpleasant. But stay away from those darn lemon and glycerin swabs. They dry out the mucous membranes, and patients dislike the taste and texture. I like to use sponge applicators dipped in warm water or used with the accompanying solution.

My advice is this: Give yourself a precious gift and do what you'd like done for someone you love and are losing. ❧

Doing the little things

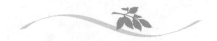

I'm an LPN who works in a long-term-care facility. Over the years, I've become more comfortable working with patients who are dying. At this point, I want to do everything I can to help these patients and their families feel cared for. What are some specific ways I can show my support and address their special needs?
—*A.R., Oregon*

I'M THRILLED THAT you're interested in providing care for patients during their final days and hours. Many health care workers shy away from these potentially powerful experiences.

The most important point to remember is that the little things really mean the most to everyone involved. For example, if you're caring for a patient who's in a coma, be sure to talk to him and encourage his family to talk to him too. Remember, he may still be able to hear even though he can't respond.

Encourage the patient's family and friends to say everything they need to say. They might want to assure him that it's okay if he wants to "cross over." Or, they may want him to know they won't abandon him if he's not yet ready to go.

Physical care is another area of importance. The dying patient needs to be turned and repositioned every 2 hours (make sure his breathing isn't obstructed). After you do this, invite family members to sit on the bed and hold the patient's hand or stroke his hair. Encourage them to do little things too, like placing a cool washcloth on his forehead, performing simple mouth care, or giving him a gentle massage. Most loved ones just want to feel useful.

But remember, there's a fine line between encouraging loved ones to participate in care and shaming them into it. If a family member isn't sure he can handle a task, don't press; he needs to do what feels right to him.

This is especially true when a patient dies. Some families want to be present for the preparation of the body; others don't. We need to help them participate as much or as little as they want.

So stay with your patient and his family but don't take over; after all, this is their experience. They just need you to help them through it.

Tricks of the trade

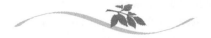

*I know you've been in palliative care for many years, and I
wonder if you'd share some of your hospice nursing "tricks." I'm
interested in caring for terminally ill patients and eager to learn.*
—*B.L., Tennessee*

CONGRATULATIONS on finding your niche. I think you'll like
the intrinsic rewards of specializing in death-and-dying nursing.

One of your major goals should be to ensure that family
members and friends aren't offended by odors—including
mouth odors, which may prevent them from sitting close to or
kissing their loved one. One clever nursing trick is using an at-
omizer to emit a fine, gentle spray of water into a semico-
matose patient's mouth. This technique provides hydration
without risk of aspiration. I use it instead of lemon and glycer-
ine swabs, which I've found are too drying. (Try one on your
own mouth to see what I mean.) You can find atomizers at
perfume counters; of course, use only brand new ones.

Another effective trick for palliative care is using multiple
pillows. This isn't new or profound, but I'm amazed at how often this technique is ignored. A dying patient will seek and
find the most comfortable position for himself—which may
appear quite *un*comfortable to staff or family members. (In
fact, sometimes nurses reposition the patient only to find that
he's turned back to the original "uncomfortable" way of lying.)

When the patient has found a favorite position, place pillows under and around those bony and achy limbs to provide
cloudlike support. Some of my dying AIDS patients may have
as many as 10 pillows cushioning them. Also, at York House
Hospice, I insist on using only 100% cotton sheets and pillow-

cases. The crisp, clean feel is more comfortable, especially for a diaphoretic patient.

An old custom I've renewed is cutting a lock of hair from a patient's head after his death. Sometimes we'll cut over a dozen locks, place each in a small envelope, then distribute the envelopes to astonished and grateful family members and friends. At the turn of the century, people commonly carried the precious hair in a locket (hence "lock") worn around their necks. You can still find them at antique markets. I like the idea and wear one myself.

Another aspect of hospice care involves final good-byes. Even if survivors were present at the moment of death, I gently offer them the chance to be alone with the body. This provides a final, private time to say those words that need to be said but weren't whispered in the presence of others. Saying good-bye at the deathbed is an extremely intimate form of leave-taking. Months later, survivors may be greatly upset if they missed the opportunity.

Finally, I offer family and friends the opportunity to help carry the body from the hospice out to the hearse. Women, rarely given the role of pallbearer, are especially eager to participate. Long after the loved one's death, survivors can still find comfort from this gesture.

These are a few techniques that I practice in hospice nursing. I hope they'll help you comfort your patients and their families.

Smelling the roses

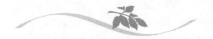

My father-in-law had chronic leukemia that became acute; he died shortly after being hospitalized. I remembered from my pediatric training that leukemia in children can be quite painful, so I kept after Dad's nurses to administer pain medication. But they hesitated because he wasn't reporting or showing signs of pain. He did receive a few injections of morphine, so I felt better and so did my husband. Do you think my father-in-law's pain was managed properly? —D.A., Wisconsin

PLEASE ACCEPT my sympathy on your father-in-law's death. It sounds as if you were a real patient advocate for him.

You're right about leukemia being painful for children. The pain results from the infiltration of leukemic cells in the long bones. (Marrow-producing cells are still active in a child's long bones.) But in adults, leukemia usually isn't terribly painful.

You say that after your father-in-law received morphine, *you* felt better. I'm wondering how *he* felt.

If you read my column regularly, you know I'm disturbed when nurses undermedicate patients who are in pain or withhold that "last" dose of morphine because they're afraid it might hasten death. But the needs and wishes of a patient without pain should be honored too.

Some patients have told me they want to be "aware" of their final moments and pain medication can interfere with that. When that's the case, you need to balance pain control with the patient's desire for awareness.

So if a patient is comfortable and peaceful, I don't medicate. Of course, if his serenity is broken by sudden changes in symptoms, I treat immediately—whether the patient is conscious or not. My patient Hilda is a good example.

A feisty lady who'd lived alone most of her life, Hilda re-fused treatment for her liver cancer and bravely struggled to stay in her little house. One day, she was brought to the hospi-tal after collapsing in her rose garden. She was close to death — but, amazingly, pain-free. Two elderly ladies from her church kept watch as Hilda lay quietly, unconscious and apparently at peace.

Then one evening Hilda began to moan through the coma. Her brow was furrowed and she grew restless. She cried out while being turned and bathed. I jumped for the telephone to inform her physician and get an order for Roxanol (morphine concentrate, 20 mg/1 ml), which I planned to administer with an eyedropper between the cheek and gum. The physician re-fused, saying "She hasn't needed anything up until now. I don't want to kill her."

"Doctor," I spoke slowly, "Hilda is going to die soon, but she's in pain now." I relayed the signs and symptoms support-ing my assessment and said I wouldn't get off the phone with-out an order for morphine. He relented.

I administered the small dose and encouraged the nurses to continue every 3 hours.

Hilda lived another 30 hours — pain-free. Two friends, a nurse advocate, and roses from her garden were by her side.

Finding contentment

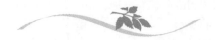

*I'm a recent graduate who's caring for an AIDS patient admitted
with vomiting and diarrhea. Those problems are being controlled
with medication. But now he's being uncooperative and rude.
I just want him to relax, settle into a daily routine, and find some
contentment. Any ideas? — C.F., Ontario*

I BELIEVE your patient is terribly affected by his diagnosis, and
that's the reason for his behavior — he's trying to come to grips
with the fact that he's terminally ill. He may even wake up
each morning wondering if today is the day he's going to die.

Second, a patient isn't suddenly better just because his
symptoms have been reversed. Your patient knows the cause of
his vomiting and diarrhea hasn't been erased. So he's probably
thinking that it's only a matter of time before he relapses.

This cycle will end only when your patient dies. He knows
that too. He feels vulnerable right now, and may simply be trying to maintain some sense of control in an uncontrollable situation. He may fear that you're attempting to control him —
this may be why he's uncooperative.

So now you need to find ways to give him some control.
(This is one of the most important lessons I've learned in my
years as a thanatologist.) Start by telling him that he's the
boss. Together, make a list of his likes and dislikes. Document
them in his plan of care, then communicate them to the nurses
on the next shift. For example, ask him what time he'd like to
be bathed — or if he even wants to be bathed. Find out from
him if he prefers his blanket folded or draped. You might offer
to give him a back rub. And when you go to the cafeteria for
lunch, ask him if he'd like you to bring anything back for him.

I think you'll both feel more content in the next few days. ✎

Talking to spirits

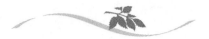

I'm caring for a terminally ill patient in an extended-care facility. She's confused and talking to people whom I don't see. I'm attentive to her pain, and she seems comfortable. But I'm concerned that her confusion might be making her anxious or frightened. Would a sedative help? —N.D., Quebec

HATS OFF to you for your compassion and advocacy. Whether or not your patient needs treatment depends on your assessment of the reasons behind her behavior. First, you need to rule out possible physical causes for why she can't communicate; for example, the discomfort of a fecal impaction or a full bladder.

Agitation is sometimes a sign of impending death. In that case, she's too anguished for counseling and requires urgent sedation. This "pain of the psyche" requires treatment just as urgently as somatic or visceral pain requires morphine. I recommend 1 to 2 mg of lorazepam (Ativan) P.O. every 4 to 6 hours for patients with terminal agitation.

But if you feel your patient is simply confused, assess the impact her confusion is having on her during these final days. If she's "pleasantly" confused, I don't advise medication. As you describe, some patients see what we do not. They talk to spirits — and enjoy the visits. ✎

Making meals memorable

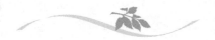

I'm a registered nutritionist working in a small hospital. Although we don't have a hospice unit per se, we have frequent admissions of terminally ill patients. I'm terribly frustrated over trying to get these folks to eat. Since you see many patients every week, do you use any special little tricks? —M.S., *Rhode Island*

YOU PROBABLY THINK that if your patient eats, he'll feel better, right? But for the dying person, the act of eating is no longer a nutritional goal; it's a social one. We should start caring more about nourishing the soul than the body.

Unfortunately, we all associate eating with living. I'd been caring for a dying woman who had worked through a lot of anger with God. Finally, she was as peaceful and accepting as anyone I'd ever seen. Her daughter came bounding into the room, tapping her mother's face and shouting, "Mama, Mama, wake up and eat the soup I brought!" The girl believed vehemently that her mother's life could be extended, if not saved, by eating the magic soup.

But cancer eats soup, too. And everything else the patient puts into his system. Malignant cells require calories. Lots of calories. Even patients who eat continue to lose weight. So we can no longer measure our success by calories or protein intake.

I've used some of the following tips that I gleaned from the Connecticut Hospice in Branford:
✦ To begin, allow patients to choose not only their food but also the size of their portions.
✦ If you cut the quantity of food in half and place it on a salad plate instead of a dinner platter, the patient may not feel so overwhelmed. Remember, we eat with our eyes, then with our

mouths. Imagine the satisfaction for a terminally ill patient to "eat everything on his plate." And make sure his tray has only one or two dishes on it, again to give the appearance of an achievable goal.

✦ Present an array of desserts on a cart, just like in a fancy restaurant. Again, serve small portions and allow the patient to take his time in choosing something yummy.

✦ For patients who require pureed food because dentures no longer fit or a tumor of the mouth prevents chewing, consider this: A method known as "reforming" takes a good old pork chop, puts it through a food processor, then reshapes it around the bone to give the appearance of a typical pork chop. This reforming helps maintain the dignity of a patient who thinks eating pureed food is demeaning.

And instead of serving an institutional scoop of mashed potatoes, have them molded into the empty skin of a baked potato. That gives the sense of original form and substance while providing nutrition and an appetizing presentation.

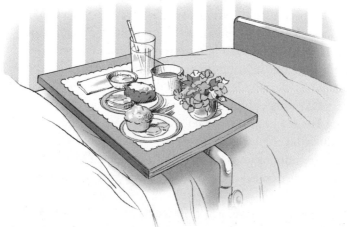

Obviously these little tricks take extra time. But I would hope you could encourage your hospital's kindhearted chef to make a dying patient's last meals a bit more meaningful. ✎

Taking the mask off

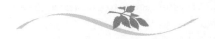

I read a column of yours in which you said you removed the oxygen mask from a dying patient's face because he wasn't struggling to breathe. When I mentioned this to one of my nursing colleagues, she said depriving a patient of supplemental oxygen is unacceptable because it would hasten his death. Can you explain your thinking?
—*N.W., Texas*

WHEN A PATIENT is in the final stages of illness and the goal is comfort care, I believe oxygen should be given only rarely because it may prolong the dying process. Oxygen isn't generally necessary for comfort. Morphine and lorazepam (Ativan) will do an excellent job of keeping a dying patient comfortable by sedating her and preventing respiratory distress.

I learned about this from an intensivist who was weaning a dying patient from a ventilator. When writing orders, he deliberately withheld an order for oxygen. He did, however, order a morphine infusion "to be titrated for comfort." This gave the nurses plenty of leeway to use their judgment if the patient began laboring to breathe.

A few weeks ago, I worked with a 62-year-old woman actively dying of lung cancer. She was comatose and appeared quite comfortable on 4 mg of morphine hourly. Her two older sisters were camped at the bedside, sharing treasured memories.

The patient was receiving 50% oxygen via a Venturi mask. Wondering if she really needed the oxygen, I gently examined her and found that her hands and feet were warm and pink, without signs of cyanosis. Her respirations were 6 per minute, deep and even.

I got the visitors some lunch, then returned 4 hours later. Reassessing the patient, I found her condition unchanged. Noticing the sisters were preparing to spend the night, I asked them how long the patient had been in the hospital.

"Three days," the older one replied. "She was just like this at home, except without a mask. She just had those little prongs in her nose."

The other sister smiled. "Helen was always vain about her looks. She wouldn't like wearing a mask."

I asked the women to join me in the hall.

"Your sister is in a deep coma and appears quite comfortable," I said. "I don't think the oxygen is doing anything to help her, and it may be prolonging the dying process. You need to hear me clearly when I say I'm not trying to hurry her along to die sooner. I just want you to have the information. Do you think she's waiting to complete any unfinished business before she dies?"

They said no in unison.

"We've been telling her that it's okay to go, that we'll be all right, but she's not going," said one.

"Do you want the mask to come off?" I asked.

"We'll talk with her son when he comes in tonight," said the other sister. "We understand what you're telling us, and we both agree."

In the end, the family decided against removing the mask; I don't know why. Perhaps Helen's son had some unfinished business of his own. But it was important to tell the family about the implications of oxygen therapy so they could make an informed decision.

In my book, this is true palliative care. ✎

Not just a pain reliever

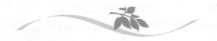

I'm caring for a nursing home resident with end-stage heart failure and pulmonary edema. He's tachypneic at 32 breaths/minute and has a look of terror in his eyes. I called the attending physician and requested small, frequent doses of oral morphine. She refused, saying, "He's not in pain, so morphine isn't indicated."

I believe a small dose of morphine would make this patient more comfortable and less panicky. Am I wrong? —*D.P., Tennessee*

NO, IT'S THE PHYSICIAN who needs a refresher course in Pharmacology 101. Morphine does much more than simply relieve pain. Because it acts as a vasodilator, it can increase cardiac output. It's also a respiratory depressant, so it suppresses the horrible drowning sensation your patient is experiencing while decreasing the respiratory drive for that next, precious breath. When oral morphine is provided for patients like yours, arterial blood gas values actually improve, proving the efficacy of morphine for dyspnea. Finally, morphine can produce a mild, but welcome, euphoria, relieving feelings of terror and panic.

I applaud you for your commitment to patient advocacy. Contact the physician again and request 5 mg of liquid morphine every 4 hours, as needed. If she still balks, go through channels to the medical director, if necessary, to get your patient the treatment he needs to relieve his suffering.

Sound judgment

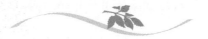

I'm an acute care nurse who occasionally works in an inpatient hospice unit. Recently, while I was administering a morphine suppository to a dying patient, the patient's wife asked me to also give him lorazepam (Ativan). I explained that her husband was minimally responsive and showing no signs of anxiety or agitation, the usual indications for lorazepam. She replied, "The other nurses do it."

In this case, I was concerned about giving another central nervous system (CNS) depressant to a patient with falling blood pressure. In general, I'm uncomfortable medicating patients just to appease family members. Is my thinking okay, or am I behaving like an acute care nurse? —*D.P., Ohio*

I THINK YOU'RE behaving like an acute "caring" nurse. In fact, in the situation you describe, you came shining through. I'm pleased that you continued to provide analgesia even though your patient was "minimally responsive." (If ever you question whether the dying person is feeling pain, please err on the side of yes.) It's just good palliative care to administer narcotics round-the-clock.

I prefer to give morphine as a concentrated oral solution rather than a suppository. For a comatose patient, you can use a small eyedropper to gently place the liquid buccally, where it's slowly absorbed.

I also like to use lorazepam, 1 or 2 mg every 4 to 6 hours, for an agitated patient. But your patient wasn't agitated, so I think you exercised good judgment in not giving lorazepam.

You replied appropriately to the patient's wife. She probably had observed other nurses giving her husband lorazepam when he was agitated and needed it. But now that he doesn't need anxiolytic treatment, morphine is the drug of choice for pain control. You can help her understand what each drug does and why lorazepam might be appropriate at one time but not another.

Telling you what drugs she thinks her husband needs is probably her way of trying to exert some control over the situation. To help her deal with the stress, encourage her to share her feelings and get her involved in care planning.

I'm sure this experience has been heartbreaking for her. She could probably use some anxiolytic therapy herself—in the form of hugs and support. ✎

Struggling with dyspnea

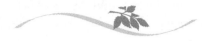

I've seen terminally ill patients suffer with dyspnea. I understand that morphine is the drug of choice for this condition. Can you elaborate? — *P.M., Michigan*

I LIKE HOW you use the word "suffer" — dyspnea is a terrifying sensation. For just a taste of what it's like, close your mouth, cover one nostril with your finger, and hold the position while you read this response.

Dyspnea occurs when the demand for oxygen is greater than the body's ability to supply it. More than 30% of terminally ill patients experience this sign. A rapid onset, say over hours or days, suggests infection or pleural effusion; gradual development may indicate tumor growth or anemia.

The most important task is to slow things down, which you can do with small, frequent doses of morphine. Robert Twycross, consultant physician with the Sir Michael Sobell House in England, suggests 2.5 mg to 5 mg every 4 hours. The route will vary according to each patient's overall condition. My preference is Roxanol, an oral liquid concentrate of 20 mg in 1 ml. It's dispensed in a 30-ml bottle with a calibrated eyedropper. (Are you still pressing your nostril shut?) I like Roxanol because it provides quick relief and is easy to titrate as needed and because oral morphine doesn't have toxic effects. Most patients with a resting respiratory rate of 30 to 40 or more will benefit nicely.

How else can you help? Don't forget standard interventions, such as administering low-dose oxygen and teaching pursed-lips breathing. Stay out of the patient's face. Don't make him talk when he needs all his energy to breathe.

You might also like to have a small table fan available. He may find the sensation of air moving across his face extremely beneficial. (For more information on dyspnea, see "Chronic Dyspnea: Controlling a Perplexing Symptom" in the May issue of *Nursing98*.)

Lastly, I like to give hand and foot rubs. This ancient relaxation technique provides superb relief and lets caregivers feel helpful.

Oh, you may release your finger. Now, imagine feeling that way for days or weeks.

Please be an advocate for dyspneic patients. They can't get relief by simply lifting a finger.

Helping hand

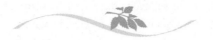

*My father, who's dying of pancreatic cancer, refuses to go to a
hospice. (He's in little pain, and he doesn't want "outside" help.)
That's fine with me and the other family members who'll help care
for him in his final days. We're wondering, though, what we can
expect. What's it like to care for a dying person?* —*J.T., Nebraska*

YOUR QUESTION IS a valid one, and my hat's off to you for
wanting to be a companion to your father in his final days. You
should feel good that you can help him do this his way. I'm
happy to give any advice that will make it easier on all of you.

To be on the safe side, ask your father's doctor to write a
prescription for a strong narcotic. Then have the prescription
filled. This may save you a panicked trip to the ED if your father suddenly wakes up in the middle of the night with excru-
ciating pain.

If you start giving him the narcotic, make sure you also give
a nightly laxative to prevent constipation. Also think about
getting a prescription for an antiemetic, such as prochlorper-
azine (Compazine) suppositories. If your father takes liquid
morphine, you may want to give him the suppository until he
adjusts to the narcotic.

Another concern for you may be his eating habits. Most
dying patients lose interest in food. You may need to keep
well-meaning friends and neighbors from forcing their culi-
nary delights on your father.

Just ask him what he'd like to eat. Be prepared for frustration. He may say, "Some rice pudding would taste good." An
hour later, after you've labored in the kitchen, you may find
that he'll take only a few spoonfuls.

He'll become progressively weaker, sleeping more and more. Take advantage of his good days. Find out what he wants to do. Ask him, every day, what he wants, then help him do it. He's ending his life, and he certainly knows what's best.

When he can't speak or rise from his bed, shift your care to keeping him clean and comfortable. Move gently; speak softly. After he slips into a coma, he'll be profoundly weak and unresponsive, but I believe he can still hear you. So keep telling him that you love him and will miss him. As his breathing becomes slower and more shallow, you can expect death within hours.

Remember to take care of yourself too. When you're feeling down, talk with other family members. Don't be afraid to cry or to ask for help when you're tired. Allowing yourself to get worn out won't be good for either of you.

You can do this. Your father trusts you, and so do I.

Safety, comfort, peace

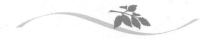

At our large medical center, several patients die each day. Do you think it's possible for anyone to die with dignity in a hospital, or can that happen only in a patient's home or a hospice?
— C.B., Missouri

I BELIEVE A dying patient's dignity can be preserved in any setting. But I'd also remind you that "death with dignity" means different things to different people. For you, it may mean being surrounded by loved ones; for me, it might mean lying unattended beneath the pine trees on my farm.

I'd submit, however, that most people require a few specific conditions for a dignified death.

✦ Whether at home, in a hospital, or in an inpatient hospice, the patient must be safe from last-minute efforts to prolong life. There's nothing dignified about being whisked away in a screaming ambulance or being poked repeatedly with a needle to find a collapsed vein.

During the dying trajectory, the focus must shift from a clinical experience ("she hasn't voided all day") to a personal and spiritual one ("Iris, we're going to take turns reading to you").

✦ The patient must be absolutely pain-free, even at the risk of double effect, which means that the amount of opioid required to keep her comfortable may also hasten her death. No patient should be denied effective pain management for any reason.

✦ The patient should be surrounded with familiar objects, sounds, and smells that comfort her. I recall an elderly woman who was delighted to receive a beautiful toy cat that was the exact replica of her own kitty. She held the stuffed animal

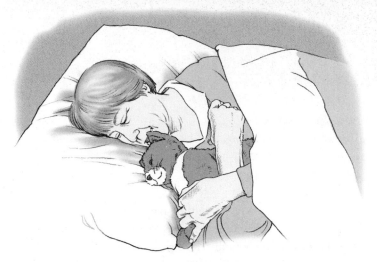

close to her heart and, for the first time in many restless nights, fell into a contented "catnap."

✦ The patient must leave the earth in her own personal style. Why exchange an elderly woman's lingerie for a hospital gown? This form of expression is integral to who she is. We all live our lives uniquely, and we should finish our lives the same way. ∞

Wondrous gift

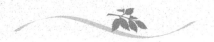

*My terminally ill niece was recently hospitalized for pain
management. I was surprised to find out that she's also receiving
physical therapy. Why are they putting her through this?*
—*A.B., British Columbia*

MAYBE YOUR NIECE requested it. You might ask her how *she*
feels.

If the message your niece has been getting from her doctors
and nurses is "nothing more can be done," she may like the
idea that something *can* be done. She may also appreciate a
scheduled event and look forward to the change of scenery
and the new faces in the halls and elevators.

I have great admiration for physical therapists. In my experience, they're a neat mix of liveliness and quiet patience. They
have wonderful talents for bringing out each patient's personal
best.

So if a terminally ill patient wants physical therapy, I see
the benefit of it. For example, home care can be much easier
for the family and other caregivers if the patient's waning abil-
ities have been maximized. Even simply learning how to
change positions in bed can be a great help to everyone. I've
had dying patients tell me how guilty they feel about waking
up an exhausted caregiver just to turn them to a more comfortable position.

Physical therapy can also restore a patient's dignity in simple ways. I recall working with a lovely woman in her 50s.
She'd been a willing and constant nurturer for her large family.
Now, although her husband and children were eager to return
all her kindness, she had difficulty being on the receiving end.

Her physical therapist had been working to help her hold a glass. Tears filled my eyes as I watched her struggle to grasp a small glass of water in her trembling hand. And my tears overflowed as I observed the restraint her family displayed by not stepping forward to hold the glass for her.

Until the patient's spirit says no, I think physical therapy can be a wondrous gift.

Honoring their wishes

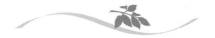

My coworker believes that terminally ill patients need to have something to look forward to each day. So every morning, she gets her patients out of bed — even if they don't want to. She also asks the doctor to write orders for physical therapy. What do you think about her philosophy? — E.L., Ohio

I BELIEVE NURSES should ask patients what *they* want, then honor those wishes.

I've learned from experience that human beings know what is best for them — right up to the moment they die. Being ill, weak, and vulnerable to a nurse who does what she determines is best must be very frightening.

Your story reminds me of Eleanor, a lovely lady in her 50s who was dying of colon cancer. When I arrived at her little apartment, I saw the visiting nurse's car parked at the curb. I looked through the screen door and could only stare in disbelief at the scene inside.

The visiting nurse was standing with her hands on her hips and perspiration beading on her upper lip. The sleeves of her blouse were rolled up above her elbows.

There, in front of her, was poor Eleanor, propped up in a straight-backed chair with pillows. Her face was gray; she held a glass of water in her pale, quivering hand.

She looked exhausted.

"I got her up," the nurse said proudly.

Somehow I managed to stop staring and form the word, "Why?"

"It makes her family feel better," she said.

I quickly slid the chair over to the bed and gently lifted Eleanor into it. She died in the few minutes it took to get her positioned comfortably.

This nurse had disregarded her patient's expressed desire to be left alone. Eleanor had been unnecessarily yanked, pulled, and plunked into a chair at a time when she really needed a nurse who would be her advocate.

That doesn't mean terminally ill patients can't benefit from some activity. But they have to choose it. I think physical therapy, for example, is a good idea. I don't mean that a dying person should be transported to the hospital for intensive therapy. But having a physical or occupational therapist work on a specific strength exercise — such as holding a cup of tea or wiping his own lips — can be meaningful to the patient.

The important thing is to ask and, no matter what the patient says, to comply.

I believe patients deserve that kind of respect from their caregivers. ✏

Window of opportunity

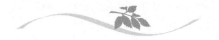

We frequently care for dying patients in our busy medical/surgical unit. Many of these patients lose consciousness quickly, before I've found time to ask about their final wishes. What can I do during these last hours to help? —R.B., Ontario

GRAB THAT WINDOW of opportunity when the patient is alert enough to reply to questions about physical, emotional, and spiritual needs. Even if you can't always guarantee that those wishes will be met, at least you'll understand what's paramount to the patient.

Recently, I visited a 52-year-old man who was dying from extensive bilateral lung malignancy. When I entered the room, I found a dozen people sprawled on various chairs, stools, and a small cot. They obviously were devoted to Mr. Panella.

I found Mr. Panella sitting on the side of the bed, his legs dangling and swollen feet bare. My clinical eye moved from his cyanotic lips to the oxygen flowmeter. Ten liters/minute!

I sat gently beside him and introduced myself, adding, "I work with patients who are seriously ill. Did you want to talk about any of your concerns?"

"Well, I'm seriously ill, all right," he replied. "And my major concern is staying alive until Monday evening when my son Joseph graduates. Do you think you can help me do that?"

I glanced at the young man named Joseph, who was crying softly.

"Mr. Panella," I began. "It has been my experience that we all participate in when and how and where we leave our body, so I'd have to say some of the power rests with you."

"Good answer!" he gasped. "So, do you think I can last until Monday?"

"I think there may be a few little tricks we might use to keep you more comfortable so you're not using so much energy to breathe. Let me call the physician for some new orders and we can get you started on resting a bit."

There was a collective "thank you" from all as I excused myself.

Mr. Panella's physician started him on some albuterol and small, frequent doses of morphine for his tachypnea. Then he asked if I wanted to see Mr. Panella's chest X-ray. Peering into the view box, I saw no left lung and only a tiny portion of the right middle lobe.

"Dear heavens, how is he still alive?" I asked incredulously.

"Sheer will, my friend," said the physician. "Sheer will."

Later that evening, I went to say good-bye to Mr. Panella. It was Friday and I was off duty for the weekend. He was asleep and appeared more comfortable. Joseph was by his side.

While driving home, I sent my best powerful energy to that dear patient. Several times during the weekend I thought about Mr. Panella and his fantastic will to live for this special occasion.

Monday morning I rushed to pull up his name on the first computer I could find. He'd died during the night. We didn't have enough tricks.

I didn't think he could do it, but I'd hoped against hope that he would. I guess what really matters is that he'd shared his goal with us and allowed us to support his efforts to reach it.

This "eleventh hour" business is difficult. If you get the chance to ask what your patient wants, make doing so a priority. If he can no longer speak, ask the family about favorite pieces of music or literature and use those at the deathbed. Be respectful and encourage others to feel the sacredness of these final hours. And whisper softly in your patient's ear how honored you are to be present, even for this fleeting moment. ✎

Who's crazy now?

A physician I work with routinely orders psychiatric consults for terminally ill patients who ask her to stop aggressive treatments. Do you think that's warranted? — S.S., Ohio

NO, I THINK it's usually an indication that the physician is uncomfortable caring for a patient at the end of life. Some physicians also want to verify and document a patient's competence for legal reasons.

Recently I got a referral to see a patient terminally ill with lung cancer and liver metastasis. His physician wanted me to talk with him about going to rehab so he could get strong enough to tolerate more chemotherapy.

I found my patient lying in bed staring up at the ceiling. I introduced myself as a clinical specialist who works exclusively with people who are seriously ill, then asked if he wanted to talk about how things were going.

He simply said, "I'm fine."

I went on to say that I was terribly sorry that the cancer had gotten away from us and that I wondered what he wanted now.

"I just want to go home."

"Home to heaven or home to your house, Mr. North?"

"Both."

I mentioned that I'd read in his chart that he hadn't eaten for many days and asked if he wanted us to try an appetite stimulant.

"No.... I'm fine."

I asked if he had any questions or concerns he wanted to discuss, and he just shook his head no. But as I got to the door he said, "Joy, I've got no reason to lie to you. I'm done, and I'm fine."

I reminded him that he could ask for me if he wanted to talk, then went to write my note in his chart.

The next day, Mr. North's excellent nurse paged me. "You'll never believe what Dr. Sutherland did!" she exclaimed. "He's ordered a psych consult for Mr. North to find out why he won't eat!"

"Mr. North doesn't need a psych consult. He's not eating because he's lost his appetite and is ready to die," I said emphatically.

The psychiatrist's consultation was brief and to the point. Her note simply said that the patient wasn't suicidal, but that he was well adjusted and accepted his terminal condition.

I believe that at certain times, some terminally ill patients can benefit from psychiatry and antidepressant treatment. But it's a mistake to routinely order psych consults for patients just because they recognize and accept their condition.

This approach is a glaring reminder of how poorly some health care providers deal with death and dying. Sorrow over leaving the planet isn't an abnormal reaction requiring analysis. Most dying patients find great comfort in just being able to share their feelings with someone who's caring and empathetic.

By the way, Mr. North went home the next day with a hospice referral. ✎

.7.

Making ethical decisions

Dying on time?

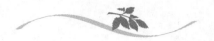

What do you think about physicians who give terminally ill patients specific time-related prognoses? I worry that the patient may feel obligated to die within that period. — *C.P., Minnesota*

I FIND IT audacious for anyone to say to a patient, "I give you 3 to 4 months." Because I firmly believe we participate in when and how we die, it really isn't useful. The following anecdote may help illustrate my point.

An oncologist told a woman who had extensive metastasis from breast cancer that she had less than 6 months to live. (The patient never asked for this information.) Three years after this death sentence was imparted, the woman met an acquaintance on the street.

"Oh my, here you are!" he blurted out. "I thought you'd be dead by now."

Smiling coyly, she extracted a yellowing newspaper clipping from her purse. It was her oncologist's obituary.

I do think it's helpful to ask the patient if she has any questions. This opens the door if she wants to know approximately how long others with this particular disease have lived. That doesn't necessarily lock her into a time frame. Many factors influence our will to live or to just let go.

I'd rather hear physicians speak within a context that's specific to a patient's life. Perhaps, "I know your daughter's planning a June wedding. The way things are progressing, I think you might want to see if they could change the date to a few months from now. I think you'll still have some energy then."

Of course, in order for a physician to suggest such an alternative, he'd have to know his patient well. Something the guy in the yellowed obituary did not. ✎

Unwelcome visitor

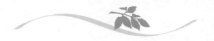

Last week, one of my terminally ill patients asked me to call her
pastor and tell him to stop visiting. When I asked why, she refused
to answer, so I never called. Did I do the right thing?
— *K.Y., Arizona*

I WOULD HAVE told the pastor about the patient's request and
explained that I tried to learn why but was unsuccessful. Your
patient may have felt uncomfortable divulging the reason, but
she was asking you to speak for her. Probably she was afraid to
tell him herself for fear of offending him.

I take patient requests at face value; I don't ask for explana-
tions. But honoring a request can be difficult when it involves
excluding people, especially well-meaning clergy.

From time to time, these individuals come to our hospice
offering to pray with our AIDS patients. I invite them in and
ask about their beliefs regarding AIDS.

Many of our patients are gay, I.V. drug abusers, or prosti-
tutes. Almost all are afraid to die. The last thing they need is
someone talking with them about burning in hell. (During my
23 years working in thanatology, I've never seen a deathbed
conversion.)

Of course, if any patient requests clergy, I comply. But our
emphasis is on spirituality, not religion. We give our patients
unconditional love and remind them that our love is minuscule
compared with the amount of God's love awaiting them.

Terminally ill patients expend a lot of energy dying. They
can't afford to waste whatever energy they have available, and
they may be highly selective when it comes to entertaining visitors. Clergy who support a dying person's beliefs are most ap-

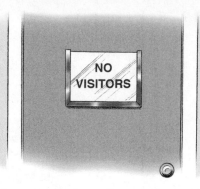

preciated. Those who drain her energy are asked to stop visiting.

I suspect your patient's pastor either said the wrong thing or failed to say the right thing. Consider trying again to discover the problem. Choose a time when you have a few minutes, sit down, take your patient's hand, and gently ask if she feels like talking about what happened to cause the pastor's "eviction."

If she wants to talk, fine. If not, show her you care, unconditionally. That may simply mean being present. Actually, that's quite adequate.

Staying silent

*I'm a gay male nurse working in a cardiac step-down unit. I'm
also HIV-positive. Three years ago, when I was first diagnosed,
I was depressed about facing a premature death. Now I'm back to
normal. I work and play hard and feel I can live for many years.
None of my coworkers — including my nurse-manager — know
that I'm HIV-positive. Am I being unethical? Should I resign?*
—*M.R., Oregon*

I DON'T BELIEVE in 'shoulding' anyone. I do find it interesting
that you write with these questions. You know as well as I that
the chance of your infecting patients or coworkers is next to
nothing. Even if you accidentally cut yourself, your professional peers would, I'd hope, observe universal precautions when
treating you. And certainly you wouldn't go dripping blood directly into the open wounds of cardiac step-down patients. So
I don't think you need to resign.

As for divulging your HIV status to your nurse-manager,
ask yourself, *Is revealing this personal information vital to my
ability to perform my professional duties?* Again, the answer is
no.

I'm not speaking unkindly when I say I'm afraid your dis-
closure wouldn't be kept confidential. And then, as they say, all
hell would break loose. As humans, we sometimes have to 'do
something' with intriguing information.

I'm not suggesting your manager would act maliciously. But
given the high level of fear associated with AIDS, even among
educated professionals, I'd say you have every ethical right to
remain silent.

Please continue to eat healthy foods, exercise, practice safer
sex, and give good nursing care to your patients.

Valley of false hope

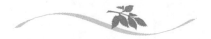

I recently cared for a patient with end-stage lymphoma in our large oncology unit. His physician told the patient and family they were out of realistic treatment options, but the patient insisted on more chemotherapy anyway. Under pressure, the physician ordered a repeat of the same drug regimen the patient had failed to respond to earlier. My colleagues and I think this was wrong. What do you say? (By the way, the patient died 1 week after receiving the drug.) — C.M., Wisconsin

I BELIEVE PHYSICIANS need to sit down and share honest and realistic expectations regarding terminal illness with their patients. Just because the patient wants a treatment doesn't mean the physician is obligated to give it.

Perhaps this physician allowed himself to be led into the valley of false hope because he had nothing clinical to offer. But the truth is he could have offered more of himself.

I've seen the effects of a gentle, caring oncologist sitting on the bed beside his dying patient. The hushed tone and sincere hand-holding were reinforced by the sense that this wise physician had nowhere else he needed or wanted to be. His patient also wanted more treatment, despite the odds. Validating the patient's desire for another round of chemotherapy, the physician said he wished with all his heart and soul that more drugs would help.

"But they just won't," he said. "You know that the last two treatments were ineffective, and I can't justify repeating them. But I'm not going to leave you. I want to help you till the end. And I promise to keep you very comfortable." Terminally ill patients are afraid of abandonment and pain, and this physician eased both fears with his promise of commitment.

Unfortunately, your patient died without the benefit of this kind of compassionate honesty.

You might argue that the patient is entitled to one last try for survival. Why not comply with his last wish?

I believe that physicians and nurses should assist with the delicate shift from "cure" to "care." Believe me, it's hard work. It's easier to smile encouragingly and say, "Okay, we'll do some more chemo," instead of sitting down, listening to the dying person's concerns, and offering hospice and the promise of a house call or two. But physicians who've taken this approach speak of a resurgence of the old feeling that drew them to medicine. Even more important, patients speak of peace and closure. ✍

Sugarcoated pain

Recently, a doctor prescribed a placebo for my terminally ill patient's pain. The doctor told me that for some patients, placebos are just as effective in relieving pain as real medication. Is that true? — R.H., *Arizona*

IN MY EXPERIENCE, when a patient says he has pain, he has pain. On occasion, however, I've been asked to speak to a patient who's having "illogical pain." (I'm still not sure what this description means, but I don't like the judgment associated with it.)

In one case, when a patient who was terminally ill with AIDS didn't respond to a typically adequate dose of an analgesic, the doctor ordered an injection of sterile water. The patient reported relief from the injection and was immediately labeled a kook. Subsequent medical and nursing care was delivered with snickers and condescending remarks.

When I visited the patient, I simply sat down with him, held his hand, and asked him if he felt like sharing with me how he was feeling about being seriously ill. He burst into tears and told me of the many sorrows in his life. He felt guilty for causing pain to his family and friends for not being who they thought he should be.

I told him the truth about the injection and said I thought talking to a psychologist would be more helpful than an injection. He gave me a big hug, grateful that there was someone to listen to him instead of sugarcoating his concerns.

8

Taking care of yourself

A real winner

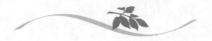

Although I care for many seriously ill patients in the course of my work (which I love), my question concerns a personal matter. Last summer, my mother died after an 8-month illness. During that time, I was her main caregiver and put my career on hold to spend more time with her. I'm still bothered by the nasty way she spoke to me the last few days that she was alive. I know she wasn't herself and I should let this go, but it nags at me. What are your thoughts?
— L. T., Michigan

DON'T GET STUCK on your mother's last words. They could have originated from pain, fear, or confusion. Focus on the real, long relationship you had with her. I'll bet it was good.

You love your work, yet you committed yourself to nursing her through the end of her life. By making this sacrifice, you provided your mother with a loving, dignified death. In my book, you're a winner. Perhaps the following story will help.

A few years ago at the Seattle Special Olympics, nine contestants, all physically or mentally disabled, assembled at the starting line for the 100-yard dash. At the gun, they started out, not exactly in a dash, but with relish, each determined to run the race to the finish and win. Moments later, one boy fell on the asphalt, tumbled over a couple of times, and began to cry. The others slowed down to look behind them, then went back. One girl with Down syndrome bent and kissed him, saying, "This will make it better." Then all nine linked arms and walked across the finish line together. Everyone in the stadium stood and cheered for several minutes.

People who were there are still telling this story. Why? Because we know what matters in life is helping others to win — even if it means slowing down and changing our own course.

Remaining vulnerable

I've been a hospice nurse for years, yet I never seem to get used to the idea of my patients dying. I always get upset and wish that I could have done more. Am I being unrealistic? —*E.W., Kansas*

NO. YOU'RE SIMPLY allowing yourself to be affected by death. Most caregivers wish they could do more for their terminally ill patients.

I've always been quick to remind caregivers that palliative care isn't passive nursing. We can always do *something* for our patients—whether it's controlling pain, managing symptoms, or lending emotional support. But sometimes, even this good advice seems trite and inadequate—even to us "experts."

I'm reminded of a patient I recently cared for. He was a handsome, high-powered, corporate executive. And was dying of cancer. He was a very proud man, a born winner and leader. He'd diligently worked his way up the corporate ladder to chief executive officer, surviving two takeovers, market changes, downsizing, and a relocation, always managing to stay on top of the ball and ensure his company's continued growth—only to be sabotaged from within by his own body.

Knowing death was inevitable, he wanted to be prepared—to be given a full report. He asked me for details about his death, which I provided honestly. He would lapse into a coma.

I admired the courage he had as he took stock of his situation and put all of his final business in order. But after talking to him, I barely made it back to my office before I was overcome by tears. Other members of the care team had similar reactions. One nurse became snappish and rude after seeing the patient. Another acted out her frustration by throwing things.

But before the day was out, we'd shared our sadness and anger with each other and exchanged long hugs. Each of us on the team knew it was safe to show that death affects us. We also know that ultimately, our vulnerability makes us better caregivers.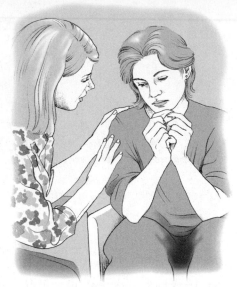

A death with dignity

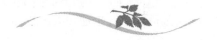

I know you have years of experience as a thanatologist. Do some deaths affect you more than others? — M.F., Pennsylvania

YES, THEY DO. In fact, a recent situation was especially moving.

It started at about 7:30 a.m. I was helping to admit Charlotte, a woman whose cancer had metastasized to her intestines. A half hour later, we were rushing her to the ICU with a rapidly dropping blood pressure and abdominal pain.

The consulting surgeon left her room after a few minutes. He shook his head as if to say, "nothing more can be done." Charlotte's doctor, a young woman on her first day of ICU rotation, beckoned to me to join the discussion.

We agreed that Charlotte needed two things: the truth and morphine for her pain.

As I took Charlotte's pale, weak hand, Charlotte's doctor leaned over the bed rail. Gently explaining that the situation was critical. Dr. Sumpkin told her that we were running out of time, that the cancer was out of control.

"Your intestine has been perforated with cancer," she said. "I'm terribly sorry, Charlotte, but you're going to die…in a few hours."

Charlotte gripped my hand, as if I could prevent death from pulling her away. She looked up at me with soft brown eyes and whispered, "Are you sure?"

"Yes," I said.

I asked her if she wanted morphine for pain, and she nodded.

Dr. Sumpkin explained that the drug could make her blood pressure drop dangerously low. "We don't want to withhold pain medication," she said. "But we want you to know what might happen, in case you want to get your family here."

I suggested that we start with a small dose. Then I quickly called Charlotte's daughter, who lived about 20 minutes away from the hospital.

When I returned to Charlotte, I took her hand again. I asked if she was afraid.

"No, not really," she answered. "In fact, you don't have to stay with me, Joy. I'm sure other patients need you."

"I'm honored to be with you," I said. "But would you prefer to be alone?"

"No."

Finally, Charlotte's daughter arrived. Dr. Sumpkin and I explained that Charlotte would live about another hour. Without hesitating, Nancy walked into her mother's room.

I put my arm around Dr. Sumpkin's shoulder. She started to tremble, then to weep. So did I.

It wasn't so much that we couldn't stop death. It was the way Charlotte was facing death — head-on, with dignity.

After a few minutes. I peered into the room. I didn't want to intrude, but I needed to check Charlotte.

Nancy was half-sitting, half-lying on the bed. They were talking, crying, laughing.

I sat down at the nurses' station. Soon, Charlotte's cardiac monitor showed ventricular tachycardia. Then nothing.

I entered the room. Nancy didn't realize her mother had died. Later, she thanked us for calling her in time.

"Mother told me she wanted to be buried in her peach dress. That's such a good color for her."

Breaking down in tears

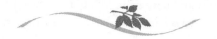

I'm a nursing student who's never seen a person die. When the time comes, I'm afraid I'll lose it and upset the patient or family. How do you do this work all the time and not break down in tears? —*F.E., Colorado*

I NEED TO REMIND you of the difference between "breaking down" and crying. If you lose control and begin sobbing, you'll also lose the ability to perform nursing duties. But that doesn't mean you should be afraid to show your emotions. I often sit quietly at the deathbed for patients and find myself crying softly. If the patient or family requires my professional skills, I simply wipe the tears and get to work. And if I feel I'm likely to "lose it," I excuse myself.

That's what happened with a beautiful patient I'll call Mrs. Watson. She was the epitome of a lady, with coiffed hair and polished nails. She called me Pussycat, and I liked her very much.

Mrs. Watson was newly diagnosed with an aggressive lung tumor that had metastasized to her spine. Frightened, she asked me to accompany her to her first radiation treatment.

As we waited for the elevator, she beckoned me close and softly asked, "Is there any hope?"

"There's always hope," I replied.

The spinal tumor was severely painful. She buried her nails deep into my palm as we positioned her on the table.

After 3 days of radiation treatment, she was still in pain, despite increasing dosages of hydromorphone (Dilaudid). Because shrinking the painful spinal tumor had been the first priority, the lung tumor had been a secondary concern. But I soon learned that it was not to be ignored.

When Mrs. Watson's condition began to deteriorate late one morning, I was slow at making the connection between the lung tumor and her severe hypoxia, confusion, and lethargy. *She must be getting too much Dilaudid,* I thought instead.

I called the attending physician for an order for naloxone. But it barely touched her respiratory depression. I pushed another 0.4 mg into her I.V. tubing. Not much response.

Then I placed my stethoscope over her right lung and heard…nothing. The tumor had rapidly replaced all three lobes. Mrs. Watson wasn't overdosed with Dilaudid; she was dying. In fact, the wonderful analgesic was all that was keeping her as comfortable as she was.

We stopped all aggressive measures and quickly converted that clinical setting into a room filled with gentle spirituality and peace.

"Mrs. Watson, it's Pussycat," I said.

"Oh, Pussycat," she weakly replied. "Don't fuss now; it's going to be all right."

I steered her husband, son, and brother close to the bed, managing to hold back tears. Then I excused myself. Ducking into the nearest stairwell, I cried hard.

She was so elegant in her suffering and dying. In the midst of her leave-taking, she'd graciously invited me in.

Becoming a better caregiver

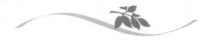

In your writing, you come off as a strong person who doesn't let death affect her. How do you do that? I feel so angry and frustrated when I can't help a terminally ill patient.—*A.T., Mississippi*

I KNOW WHAT you mean. I guess sometimes I forget how tough this work can be.

But I can't forget one especially heavy week. I was feeling frustrated over two patients in particular. Both were retired military men with nice wives and wonderful sons and daughters-in-law.

Both had diseases that would fell them by the summer's end.

One gentleman, the major, had been Army. The other, a colonel, was Air Force. Each had spoken of adroitly evading "the bullet with my name on it" during numerous battles. Perhaps that was the irony—that, in the end, they would die *this* way.

I was terribly affected by their plight, their pluck. And frustrated by the inability of modern medicine to do anything to help them.

In the past, I'd been quick to remind caregivers and patients that there was always something that could be done, in the way of palliative care, emotional support, and pain and symptom management. But now, somehow, that all seemed so trite to me.

I liked these men, and their courage in the face of death was endearing. Throughout the day, I traveled back and forth, from the major to the colonel, listening to their stories, watching them organize their "troops" for the leave-taking.

The final blow for me was when each soldier, within an hour of the other, asked me to give him specific details about his death.

One would hemorrhage, the other slip into a coma.

I hurried down the back stairs, barely reaching my office before the tears started coming.

One of our counselors, a trained observer with a big heart, risked asking, "Are you okay?"

And I risked responding, "No, I'm not okay."

John patted and comforted and talked, with a lump in his own throat, about how death gives meaning to life and how we wouldn't appreciate sunshine without rain. Then we both laughed over him reminding me, the "expert," about how death affects us.

Later, during our team conference, I saw the oncologist assigned to the two dying men act out his frustration and disappointment. He cussed and growled and made disrespectful comments until I moved my chair beside his and shared my own sadness.

It took a few minutes to sink in, but he got it.

We regrouped and worked together to make care plans for the terminally ill patients for whom nothing more could be done.

Just before we left the conference room, I gave that strong oncologist a big hug. At that moment, each of us on the team knew that it was safe to show how much death affects us.

And that vulnerability is what makes us much better caregivers.

Help for beleaguered staff

*As the ICU clinical coordinator at a large university hospital, I'm
concerned about my nursing staff. Several terrific nurses recently
left for personal reasons, leaving the remaining staff frazzled and
demoralized. What can I do to boost their spirits?*
—*F.E., California*

CONGRATULATIONS on taking a proactive approach to your
unit's morale problem. Too often we wait for the flu or an in-
jury to justify making a fuss over ourselves and our colleagues.
This isn't a judgment; I've done it myself. But I think it's
healthier for us to come out and ask for some TLC when we
need it. So here are some suggestions that might give you and
your staff a lift.

First, consider seeking out someone in the hospital who's
experienced in guided imagery. This wonderful relaxation
technique can be a great "gift" to stressed employees. Find a
small, quiet room and have the guided imagery leader conduct
a 10- or 15-minute session there — undisturbed — every week.
I think you'll find nurses will feel less tense on routine days
and better able to bounce back more quickly on wild ones.

Another recommendation is for administration to pay for a
massage therapist to come in a few times a month. Even a 10-
minute massage can relax a stressed-out nurse's back, neck,
and shoulders. Your staff might want to pay for more frequent
sessions out of the unit's "sunshine fund." (Many nurses regularly contribute to this kind of fund to buy flowers for ill or injured coworkers.)

My last suggestion may seem a bit odd, but a recent experience reminds me that a pet visitation program for patients can
have a magical secondary benefit for the staff. Recently, a

young woman was admitted to our ICU in critical condition due to fatty liver disease from pregnancy. Her unborn infant had been dead for 2 days and had to be delivered immediately. The situation was terribly sad for our staff, most of whom are young mothers themselves. I offered to speak with Greta about the loss of her baby, but she declined.

The following morning I once more offered my services, which were quietly refused. I noticed a photograph of a large, golden dog with a Frisbee in its mouth. When I asked about the dog, Greta launched into a sweet monologue about "Scooter" and how much she loved and missed her. I asked if she thought she could manage a visit from the dog. She beamed and said she'd call her husband right away.

The visit was semiraucous, but no harm was done. Greta brightened. Her appetite improved and we had two good grieving sessions while looking over birth photographs and sharing shattered hopes and dreams over her dead daughter.

But Greta wasn't the only beneficiary. That one visit from Scooter delighted the ICU staff, providing a moment of relief from a heart-wrenching situation.

Exotic getaway

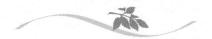

I'm on leave from my job as an OR scrub nurse. My husband of 37 years died during mitral valve replacement surgery 6 months ago. We did everything together, and now I can't get on with my life, especially work. I know this sounds strange, but I just want to go off to a foreign country and live in a monastery — not as a nun, but maybe as a cook or housekeeper. Did you ever hear of someone in my situation doing this? —*S.A., Wisconsin*

I USUALLY SUBSCRIBE to the adage "There's no *right* way to grieve, only *your* way." But I fear that in this case, "*your* way" is to run away, as if you could simply leave your grief and loss behind. Because this illusion can be powerful, I advise survivors to avoid making major life changes, such as selling a house or moving to another town, during the first year of grief.

Your desire to leave your homeland and dramatically change your lifestyle has me concerned. If you'd always dreamed of living in another country and devoting yourself to others, I could see how your husband's death could release you to pursue that dream. But your admitted difficulty in adjusting to your husband's death is a warning flag that tells me you'd probably benefit from speaking with a therapist.

Under the circumstances, I'm not surprised that you can't face returning to the OR. But I'll bet your desire to help others can be fulfilled in many ways, even nursing in another specialty.

Please ask someone in social services, pastoral care, or psychiatry to refer you to a compassionate counselor. After one year, honestly look at your life. If you still need to go away, then you'll know it's out of a true calling, not a move made out of grief and illusion. ✎

Who'll care for me?

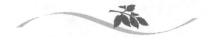

Working as a home hospice nurse, I have a busy life. I'm also a widow whose only child is grown and living across the country. Lately I've started thinking about what would happen to me if I developed a terminal illness. I'm fine now, so I'm not sure what's provoking this preoccupation with death. Are my thoughts normal? —*B.H., British Columbia*

I DON'T CONSIDER your thoughts to be a "preoccupation"; I think reflecting on the inevitable is healthy. But is it "normal"? No.

You're actually quite exceptional. Most of us humans don't *really* believe that we're going to die. If we did, we'd live our lives very differently.

You're probably identifying with your patients and their circumstances. This isn't unusual among palliative caregivers. Do you recall thinking during nursing school that you had whichever "disease of the week" you were learning about in class? If you're like most of us, it didn't matter if it was leprosy or myasthenia gravis — you had it!

Most likely, many of your coworkers have similar concerns; it comes with the territory. Even someone with a more extensive support network available than you have may worry about burdening her family if she were sick or dying.

Consider creating a support group of friends, especially nurses, who share your concerns on this subject. You could then establish a "code of care," promising each other to provide nursing care should the need arise. This way, each member of the group will know that one of the gang will be there to ensure dignified, competent care. You might meet monthly at one another's homes to discuss specific fears while testing

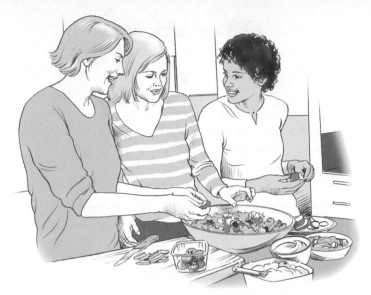

dessert recipes or working for a favorite charity. In the process, you'll develop trust and devotion.

Finally, try strengthening your bond with your child, despite the distance between you. It's well worth the investment — not only for the future, but also for the simple joy of the here and now. ❧

Off to Africa?

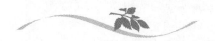

I'm in my 50s and have been an RN for many years. I like the people I work with and most of my days are satisfying. But lately I've been wondering if I could do more to help my fellow man. Do you ever feel like joining a health care team that works in Africa and leaving all the trappings of your current life behind?
—D.C., Ontario

TO BE PERFECTLY honest, yes—I do occasionally have those same musings, especially when I read about the horrible situation in sub-Saharan Africa and the growing AIDS epidemic on the continent. But I could never speak for you about this kind of life-changing decision. Some people who join relief organizations describe their work as the most rewarding labor of love that they'd ever experienced. Others report an exhausting, overwhelming time during which they, too, became ill with parasites or fevers and couldn't even care for themselves, let alone a clinic full of starving patients.

Only you can make the decision that's right for you. A good way to start is by talking with people at the international programs such as Doctors Without Borders, to learn exactly what's involved.

And remember, you don't have to go overseas to serve your fellow man—you can find many opportunities for rewarding volunteer work in your own backyard.

For me, in the here and now, I feel I'm having a positive effect on many of my patients as they finish the story of their life. I continue to believe that there are no coincidences and that I'm supposed to be with Mrs. Scott in Room 322. So when I enter her world, I treat it as a sacred experience, an opportunity to give using my skills and training, as well as a chance to show compassion. And that's immensely rewarding too.

Like all of us mortals, you too must die. Make sure your deathbed mutterings aren't full of "should haves" and "would haves." Instead, depart this world like a queen leaving a banquet table, filled with a life well lived. ✎

Build trust

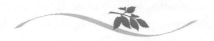

One of my patients, a woman with breast cancer, is constantly pushing her call light. But whenever I check on her, she wants something silly — "A box of tissues, please, dear" or "open the window shade, please dear." I don't want to sound unkind, but this patient is driving me crazy. What can I do? — N.G., Mississippi

YOU AREN'T UNKIND, perhaps just unaware of her real needs. This patient is frightened — scared to death, in fact. You don't mention her prognosis or if she's newly diagnosed, but cancer is scary. Her petty requests are simply ploys to get you into her room.

She may be unwilling to risk rejection by simply asking you to sit with her for a few minutes. I know one patient who made that request, only to hear, "You're not the only patient I have, you know." He never asked again.

I recall caring for a 38-year-old woman who'd had both breasts removed within a year and was hospitalized again because the cancer had spread to her liver. Her husband rarely visited, bill collectors harassed her by phone, and her teenage children never even sent get-well cards. She was on her call light constantly, but the ploy backfired — the nurses ignored her. Then they felt guilty and angry because they realized they shouldn't be treating a patient that way.

I called a conference around the woman's bed and asked her to tell us what we were doing right and wrong. During this discussion, she confessed to feeling lonely, abandoned, and isolated. She just wanted us to pay attention to her.

We agreed to be more helpful. We started by chipping in and buying her an inexpensive watch. Then the nurses assigned each other 15-minute "shifts." One nurse would stop in

Insights on death & dying

her room at least every 15 minutes to see if she needed anything. Of course, if she needed something special, she could press her call light anytime.

After only 4 hours, she settled down. She now had a sense of control, and her biggest need was being met.

The next day, in another bedside conference, we agreed to extend our shifts to 30-minute intervals. During the next few days, we gradually lengthened the time. She could still press her call light whenever she wanted something special, but she didn't seem to need to do that as much anymore. She'd begun to trust us.

Perhaps you might try this with patients who demand special attention. You'll all be happier.

Letting go

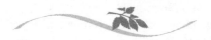

We have about 100 deaths a year at our nursing home. The staff members are devoted to the residents, but they don't seem to have an opportunity for closure. What's the best way to acknowledge these deaths? —*L.M., Georgia*

FOR YEARS, I've organized an annual ceremony to help the staff with closure. At first, we called it Balloon Day. We'd write patients' first names or initials on the balloons, then let the balloons go. That seemed like a tangible way for the staff to let go of patients who'd died during the past year.

But because balloons pollute the environment, we no longer do this. Instead, we now plant inexpensive pine tree seedlings, which can be purchased in large quantities. Unlike the balloons, the seedlings help the environment.

As we plant the trees, we speak a few words of respect or read a brief poem. We still feel as if we're letting go of the patients and any lingering feelings of attachment, so we're ready to move on.

Annual memorial services can be helpful too.

We make a list of all the patients who've died during the past year. Then we write personal letters to the next of kin, inviting them to attend and to bring along other relatives or friends if they'd like. We always have a full church.

The service is ecumenical, with a rabbi, priest, and minister officiating. A few musical selections and readings are given, as well as short sermons from the clergy. A local florist donates a huge flower arrangement, which is placed near a silver bowl that contains burning incense.

After each nurse reads her list of deceased patients, the list is dropped into the bowl. It burns and mixes with the smoke that rises to the ceiling.

This is a terribly moving ceremony that's welcomed by both staff and family.

Following the ceremony, we hold a reception. This is a wonderful time to reunite families with nursing staff. Once again, they share stories, good and bad memories, a few tears, laughter, and a lot of hugs.

Everyone is glad he or she risked grieving again and taking a step toward healing.

Believe me, your staff members will thank you for a ceremony like this. Afterward, they'll feel rejuvenated and ready to continue giving their best to their patients.

Games patients play

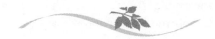

I have a terminally ill patient who makes me so mad I'm at my wit's end! She won't do a thing for herself, and when I try to assert myself, she threatens to faint or vomit. Then I feel so guilty I end up doing whatever she wants. I know she's manipulating me, but what can I do about it? —L.R., Alberta

SOUNDS AS IF this lady is trying to see how far she can push you. You're understandably reluctant to show your anger or hurt her feelings because she's already suffering enough. So you end up playing along with her.

Nurses get satisfaction from being needed, and this patient is certainly happy to be needy. What can you do? Instead of trying to control her behavior, you can help her get in touch with what she truly needs.

If I were her nurse, I'd simply ask her what she wants. She'd probably say, "to get out of this hospital."

That would give you a staring point. Then, you could help her identify what *she* can do to make that happen. Maybe it means helping with her own bath, feeding herself, or walking from the bed to the chair. Make suggestions. Get her family and other staff members involved. The secret is continuity— everyone working toward the patient's goal.

Sure, she'll have little setbacks. You need to be patient and kind but firm. Encourage her efforts, and don't forget to pat her—and yourself—on the back.

Remember, for a long time she got what she wanted by being dependent. So be prepared to accept whatever she can accomplish, even if she never reaches the level of independence you'd like. ✎

Insights on death & dying

Home-grown advice

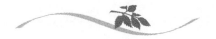

As a physical therapist, I sometimes work with terminally ill patients who could die within weeks. Sometimes I feel frustrated to think that all their hard work won't amount to much. How can I get more satisfaction out of the work I do? —J.H., Maryland

MAYBE THIS STORY will help. Last spring, I had the honor of caring for John Selman, a 78-year-old farmer who'd been admitted to the hospital with advanced prostate cancer. His nurses asked me to see him because he was depressed and in severe pain.

I found Mr. Selman slouched in a wheelchair outside the physical therapy (PT) department, dressed in a gray sweatsuit. His demeanor was as dull as his outfit. I introduced myself and asked if we could talk about his pain.

"I ain't no crybaby, Miss, but I'm hurtin' pretty bad," he confessed.

So my first order of business was to review his analgesic regimen and modify it. I settled him back in his room and called his physician, who revised her orders based on my suggestions. By mid-afternoon, Mr. Selman was pain-free and ready to talk some more.

"I see from your chart that you're a farmer," I said. "Do you have beef or dairy cows?" That's all it took. He spoke for an hour about his huge farm, which had been in his family since 1750.

"George Washington was around then, Miss," he beamed. And then he spoke seriously, symbolically. "My daddy told me a man has only 50 plantings in his life. I've had 65 plantings, so I guess I'm on borrowed time."

I told him about the many drugs available now for pain and gave him my word I'd work with his physician to keep him comfortable.

The next day, I found him getting bathed and dressed for PT — again in a sweatsuit, which the aide had suggested for convenience. But Mr. Selman just didn't look comfortable in it. So I asked him what *he* wanted to wear.

"What I've worn every day of my life, Miss. Them blue pants and shirt there."

Clothes are an extension of our personality. This man had never worn a sweatsuit in his entire life! Putting on the blue pants and shirt required just a bit more effort from the aide, but it paid off. Mr. Selman participated willingly in PT and began to make progress. He'd set a goal for himself: To get back to the farm.

"I know I'm going home to the graveyard," he told me, "but I want to climb up on the tractor one more time."

I felt he was losing precious spring days being in the hospital. So I worked with his family, hospice, and a private physical therapist to get Mr. Selman home sooner than scheduled. He was as well as he was ever going to be.

Our last conversation was a mixture of tears, laughter, and lessons. I thanked him for our talks and asked what he'd teach me that I could pass on to my next patient.

"I don't know much about stuff like that. Maybe, it would be that if you love what you do, the work ain't hard."

I'm passing his wise words on to you. I think Mr. Selman would be pleased if you took them to heart.

Index

Patient/family advocacy
(continued)
  pain management, 7-8,
    187-189, 204-206, 214-215,
    222-224
  pet visits, 195-196
  postmortem care, 202-203, 213
Patient management, 208-238.
    See also Palliative care.
  activity and exercise, 231-234
  agitation, 217, 222-224
  bedside manner, 208-213
  comfort measures, 208-213. *See
    also* Pain management.
  death with dignity, 229-230
  dyspnea, 225-226
  final wishes, 235-236
  nutrition, 218-219, 227-228
  oxygen administration,
    220-221, 225
  physical therapy, 231-234
  sedation, 217
  tricks of the trade in, 212-213
Perinatal death
  grieving for, 89, 151-153
  mementos of, 65, 89
Pets
  concerns about, 109-110,
    145-146, 195-196
  death of, 80-84
  visits by, 195-196, 258
Photographs, of stillborn
    infants, 65
Physical therapy, 231-234
Physicians
  communication with, 159-160
  grieving by, 72-73
  insensitive/remote, 197-200
  patient dumping, 199-200
  role in hospice care, 159-160
  treatment withdrawal/refusal,
    182-186, 237-238. *See also*
    Treatment, withdrawal/re-
    fusal of.
Pillows, 209, 212-213

Pink wheelchair syndrome,
    190-192
Placebos, in pain management,
    246
Positioning, for comfort, 209,
    212-213
Possessions, comfort provided by,
    52-53, 69, 100
Postmortem care, 142-143,
    202-203, 213
Prefuneral ceremonies, 87
Prognosis
  coping with, 29-30, 119-120
  time-related, 240
  truthful discussion of,
    29-30, 120
Prolongation of life, inappropri-
    ate, 5-6, 8, 182-186. *See
    also* Treatment, withdrawal/
    refusal of.
Psychiatric consult, for treatment
    refusal, 237-238

Q
Questions. *See also* Communica-
    tion.
  "Am I dying?", 29-30, 120
  asking "right" questions,
    22-23, 46

R
Regrets, 178-179
Relationships, strengthening of,
    11-12. *See also* Family.
Religious beliefs
  clergy visits, 241-242
  ethical aspects, 241-242
  talking about, 26-28
Respiratory support, 220-221,
    225-226
Role changes
  for adult children, 102-103, 116
  for widows and widowers,
    20-21
Roxanol, 225. *See also* Morphine.
  for dyspnea, 225-226